Praise from Early Readers of
Caregiver Confidential

"I think your book is amazing and right on point. I expected it to be a bit different, but it's just how I think a book should be written from the caregiver's point of view—its effect on them. I especially enjoyed it because I knew so much about it."
—Kristin Einberger, Consultant for Early Memory Loss

"I have read your manuscript; in fact, I found it so interesting that I completed it in just a few days. After reading your accounts of how you felt at various times and occasions, I could relate to that so many times. It was very interesting to hear how you coped with situations as they arose. I have been reading many blogs online about caregiving, and they are typically about caring for parents or other relatives—not so much about spouses. I must say that it is very different. I appreciate your candor and honesty."
—Karin Wasell, caregiver for her husband with Alzheimer's

"Amazing story of love, persistence, stamina, and a complex array of emotions across the points of tension that characterize the dramatic change in the anatomy of a relationship. An excellent read, written by an honest and skillful reporter/storyteller."
—Helen McDermott, family caregiver

Caregiver Confidential

Stories of Living with My Husband's Alzheimer's Disease

Cheri J. Bailly-Jacobs

Alta Pearl Press

Printed in the United States of America.

Alta Pearl Press
1370 Trancas Street, #381
Napa, California 94558

alzheimerscaregiverconfidential.com

Some individuals' names have been changed to protect their privacy. Those pseudonyms, listed in alphabetical order, are Bernie, Chris, Dan, Evelyn, Elizabeth, Gina, Isabella, Joan, Michael, Patrick, Sheila, and Sharon.

Caregiver Confidential: Stories of Living with My Husband's Alzheimer's Disease / Cheri J. Bailly-Jacobs — 1st edition.
ISBN 978-1-7347473-1-7 print
ISBN 978-1-7347473-0-0 ebook
Library of Congress Control Number: 2020904691

Dedication

To the memory of my husband, Robert N. Jacobs, who encouraged me to write about both of our lives as they were affected by his Alzheimer's disease. His consistent willingness to try all of the suggestions I made during his illness was a gift to me. Our attempts to adapt to his illness—some successful, some not—gave us both a higher quality of life while we lived with the decline of his body and the destruction of his mind, but never his spirit.

Acknowledgments

I want to thank my initial editor, Alison Owings, for her patience and encouragement. She helped me replace my succinct business writing style with a storytelling voice that included more description and detail. Her view of the importance of telling about a caregiver's experience with Alzheimer's encouraged me to keep writing.

I owe a debt of gratitude to the members of my writing group: Kathryn Winter, Paulette Litz, and Tammy Glathe. They never tired of reading another draft of the many chapters I had to revise again and again.

Professionals in the field of mental health and dementia provided me with the support and advice I needed at just the right time. Listed in order of when they came into the project, they are Lynne L. Ehlers, Ph.D.; Kristen Einberger, B.A., Memory Loss Consultant; and Gail Frizzell, BC-DMT, LCSW.

I send my special appreciation to readers who critiqued the manuscript in its many stages: Adelle DiGiorgio, Alla Crone-Hayden, Diane Gallaher, Helen McDermott, Thomas McDermott, Judy Nystrom, Sylvia Radabaugh, Patricia Rodgers, Joan Simpkins, and Karin Wasell.

I want to thank my family and the many friends who offered support and maintained interest in the project even when they thought it might be finished — but wasn't.

Extraordinary thanks to Muriel Rogers for being a diligent and astute copywriter and for bringing creativity to the challenges of book design. Her coaching me through the tough times kept me working for a better book when I just wanted to get to the end.

Contents

Contents (continued)

Introduction

My husband, Bob, was the healthiest man I knew. In spite of that, just before he turned 75, his struggle with dementia began, and I became his caregiver.

Initially, I was alone in caring for him and unprepared. I frequently felt frustrated, angry, and sad. Throughout my years of caregiving, I never found a book that honestly described those feelings as typical for a caregiver. I wanted to understand all the feelings I had, especially as his disease progressed and caregiving became more time-consuming and problematic. I didn't think about writing my own stories, for others to read, until sometime after he passed away.

In 2002, Bob had received the diagnosis of Mild Cognitive Impairment (MCI) that was to transform our predictable and pleasant life. I was self-employed and busy with my human resources management career, having started a consulting business to assist small organizations in the San Francisco Bay Area.

Bob was retired from an estate planning career and ran all aspects of our personal life, including all financial matters. I consulted with my clients, frequently from my home office, and taught business courses at local community colleges.

In the early stages of his disease, I sometimes went to my computer in the early evening and wrote about a frustrating incident in caring for him that day. At my computer, I discovered I could write an anecdote and vent all the feelings I had from the caregiving day. A typical and particularly upsetting example was losing him in the grocery store when I was quickly trying to buy food for our next week's meals. Expressing my frustrations at the computer somehow opened a space for me to find more energy and patience for the next day.

It never occurred to me to read those stories to a friend, but I sometimes read them to Bob. I would approach him as he relaxed in the living room. "I just finished making a story out of what happened today. Would you like me to read it to you?"

He always responded with an enthusiastic "Yes."

When I finished reading, I would check with him to see if my written version of the incident made him feel exposed, as if I weren't protecting his privacy. He seemed somewhat surprised that I would even think that and instead offered a compliment. "I think it's great that you're doing this. You write it just like it happened."

Then he would give me a big hug. It seemed to me that Bob appreciated hearing about himself almost the way a child likes seeing himself in a video. In turn, I loved his reactions. His encouragement about the story did not, however, spur me to write another one the next day. That motivation came when I next needed to express my exasperation and frequent anger.

Eventually, I told a few friends about my writing. They often replied, "Oh, you should keep a journal. It would be a great way to keep track of what's happening and would be good therapy for you." I rejected their well-meaning advice. Writing up an anecdote from time to time was healthy for me, but I couldn't think of anything worse than living through a day as his caregiver and then using my free time in the evening to recap everything in a journal. I wanted to spend the last part of each day crawling into bed and reading a novel that took me far away from my caregiving reality.

As honest as I could be in the stories about my daily frustrations, I never talked to Bob about how much I didn't want to be a caregiver for anyone. We had always talked about everything, but I couldn't burden him with the feelings of disappointment I had about spending my last years with him as his caregiver. I knew he probably also had feelings of loss, as the disease took over his abilities to do the many activities he had treasured.

Sometime after Bob died, I started thinking about the anecdotes I had written. I wondered if I could develop those into chapters of a book that might help other caregivers. Nevertheless, my grief kept the door closed to the idea.

Then a friend asked me to join a small writers' group she was putting together. I thought, here's my opportunity to further explore my feelings when I was a caregiver to Bob. I joined the group and found that the requirement of producing a "chapter" twice a month was the discipline I needed.

In preparing for the group meeting, I realized that the more experiences I wrote about, the more I remembered. My fellow writers were encouraging, and I began to recall how I had searched for a book that concentrated on the caregiver, rather than the decline of their loved one. I would have appreciated reading the honest reactions and feelings of a partner/caregiver while I was actively caregiving.

Finally, in 2015, I made a commitment to develop the stories into a book. It was a scary prospect for several reasons. My previous writing experience was focused on business communication that included policies, reports, and proposals to other business professionals. I had not written stories of any kind for others to read. My recently retired friends were taking trips, signing up for college courses for fun, and even playing bocce ball. Writing a book during my retirement years was not something I had ever dreamed about.

Then I recalled what I had learned from a social worker while participating in a caregiver support group: The person with the diagnosis and the caregiver each lives through the decline from a dementia disease, but each has a unique experience of it. I certainly had my nine years of unique experiences I could share, and then I recalled Bob's enthusiasm for the anecdotes I had read to him. That, more than anything, gave me the confidence and courage to tell my stories.

Part One

Entering the World of Alzheimer's

CHAPTER 1

Who Wants to Be a Caregiver?

My husband, Bob, received a diagnosis of Mild Cognitive Impairment (MCI) in 2002. That pronouncement said there was something wrong with his brain. It was a shock to our peaceful life, but I was relieved that the professionals who evaluated him didn't say Alzheimer's disease. Nonetheless, our lives were to change soon and regularly going forward.

We didn't talk much about what we would do next. As a business consultant, I frequently worked for companies where I was responsible for preparing the plan for a project. I thought Bob would assume I would do the same for his health situation. As much as I always liked having a plan for most challenges, I wasn't ready to make plans for anything yet.

Only a week after learning about the MCI diagnosis, Bob surprised me when he found an announcement in the local paper about an informational meeting about memory loss. I was pleased he was already thinking about ways we could begin to find resources.

We attended the session sponsored by Redwood Caregivers Resource Center and led by a social worker named Evelyn. At the end of the meeting, she invited us to explore the possibility of joining dual support groups. One group was for individuals with a form of dementia and the other for their family caregiver. We both had previous experience participating in a support group and knew it would be a group of people with struggles or concerns in common who, through sharing of their stories, could provide each other with encouragement and advice. A counselor or therapist usually acted as the leader of the group, assisting the discussion and assuring that participants felt safe to speak. I looked at Bob to see his reaction to her invitation. The smile on his face indicated the openness I was hoping for. I breathed a silent sigh of relief, feeling the beginning of a plan to address our new situation.

Later, Evelyn called me with instructions to drive to a nearby town the following week to meet with her and another social worker who would interview us for the support groups. "We wouldn't want to take you to the cancer ward right after you'd received a cancer diagnosis," was her explanation for the interviews. I didn't quite know what she meant, but I felt like she was trying to be careful, since Bob's diagnosis was so new to us.

A few days later, I drove us from Napa through the countryside to the town of Sonoma to attend the interviews. Driving through the vineyards brought back many romantic memories of picnicking and bike riding in our early days in the Napa Valley shortly after our marriage.

I was brought back to reality when we arrived in the town, and I parked the car near the Senior Center for the meeting. I said to Bob, "This is it, sweetie." He didn't move until I asked him to get out of the car. I was not yet used to his needing directions for everyday actions.

"Should I take my jacket?" he asked.

"Yes, take your jacket," I answered. "You can always take it off if you get too warm." He seemed relieved to have the decision made for him. Hand in hand, we walked through the parking lot and made our way to the front door.

I could see two women waiting at the Center entrance. I shook hands with Evelyn first. She quickly introduced us to her colleague, Sharon. "Hello, you must be Cheri and Bob?" Sharon said. She was middle-aged and gracious like Evelyn. I liked that they were mature women, with years of experience in their field. "Were the directions okay?" Evelyn wanted to know. Their concern reassured me too. It felt like a maternal arm had gone around my shoulders, and I started to feel at ease.

They led us into the building and through a large, institutional room with big tables, probably meant for group meals. I was pleased when we were invited into a smaller, more intimate place where we all met together for about 30 minutes. Evelyn asked us to tell them about our situation. I briefly conveyed the story of my noticing changes in Bob's memory, his frustrations with managing any detail, especially appointments, and the subsequent MCI diagnosis. As I spoke, he sat calmly, hands folded, listening courteously. I explained that we learned that MCI could advance into a type of dementia, but nothing was for sure. Whatever it might turn out to be, we were researching resources now and for the future.

When I reached that point in our story, Sharon got up from her chair, looked at Bob and asked, "Bob, would you like to come with me so we can talk together in another room?" Bob followed her like a puppy. It was sweet to see him still be the gentleman that I had always known, but it concerned me a bit that he was so compliant with a stranger. He barely glanced at me as he left the room.

I understood that I was to stay with Evelyn. I liked the idea that I would have time alone with her and wouldn't have to worry that what I said might embarrass Bob.

Evelyn started our interview by telling me that Sharon would be determining if Bob's cognitive abilities were similar to the others in the support group. She explained that it might be depressing for him if the limited capabilities of others gave him a devastating picture of his future. Her explanation helped me understand her earlier comment about visiting a cancer ward. Then she pulled out a packet of papers and began asking me for contact information: name, address, phone, etc.

Soon her questions turned to my observations about Bob's behavior and what difficulties he was having. "When did you notice that Bob was having difficulty with his memory? Is he having trouble with financial information? Can he still do personal care—showering and dressing? What other kinds of problems is he having?"

I liked that Evelyn was asking my opinion about these matters. The answers to these questions were easy for me. I knew more than anyone else about Bob and observed him regularly, especially when he wasn't watching. And I liked that, with Bob now out of the room, I could be frank. And I was.

Then Evelyn began to turn the spotlight on me. "Do you find that you are feeling stressed in your role as a caregiver? Do you have any relief from your caregiver responsibilities?" I didn't have ready answers to these inquiries—

Evelyn had caught me off guard. I thought we were going to be talking solely about Bob. Her reference to me as Bob's "caregiver" surprised me. I didn't think of myself that way. I knew the recent diagnosis of MCI probably meant I would be taking on more responsibility for his appointments and keeping track of his medical information. But the word caregiver had the feel of a full-time nurse.

Evelyn, looking down at her paperwork, asked a few more questions, which I answered the best I could. I felt unprepared to talk about many of the subjects with much detail.

Then I realized the most crucial question for me was not on her list, and despite not wanting to seem rude, I interrupted her. "Aren't you going to ask me first if I want to be Bob's caregiver?"

Evelyn seemed stunned and didn't respond to my question. I didn't know what to say in that silence. Finally, having gathered her thoughts, she said, "Well, no one has ever asked that before, but it does make sense that we should ask. I guess we've just made some assumptions about the spouse of a person with memory issues. We'll have to think about that."

She turned back to her questionnaire, ready to continue, but the reality of our new state of affairs began to hit me. Suddenly, I blurted out, "I feel like it is presumed I will be Bob's caregiver, and no one has even asked if I want to do it."

Then I could say no more. The tears streamed down my cheeks. Bob was the love of my life, our marriage a nurturing partnership. I would do anything for him. I had been imagining I would continue as I had over the past year, gradually assuming more household responsibilities. I had already taken on bill-paying and doing more of the driving. But until Evelyn's questions, I had not realized the expectation that doing some of the household tasks for Bob might eventually mean I would be doing everything.

After my outburst, we both sat quietly for several minutes. Finally, Evelyn asked, "Can you answer the remainder of the questions?" Then she patiently waited for me to respond. I nodded my head in agreement. In another few minutes, we finished the interview, and I was in some measure back to my former self—dry-eyed and more relaxed.

Evelyn thanked me for my cooperation and then led me out to the large room where we rejoined Bob and Sharon. Bob was smiling and acting like everything was fine. Sharon explained they had completed their interview, and we were free to go. Both women walked us to the door, thanked us again for coming, and said they would contact us in a few days to let us know about joining the support groups.

Bob and I thanked them in return and walked to the car. Bob was cheerful, and as we walked, he said, "I had a really good conversation with Sharon. Did you like talking with Evelyn?" He was always good at remembering people's names. I felt confident he'd had no idea that the conversation was an assessment of his cognitive abilities. He probably considered the interview to be a get-acquainted session. I was grateful he felt no pressure to perform.

To reassure him, I answered, "Yes, it was fine," but my mind was still staggering from the sudden realization that my life was about to change in ways I never imagined. During our marriage, Bob and I talked many times about the significant difference in our ages—he was 17 years older than I—and how that might make for unexpected developments. But what had I been thinking? Since his diagnosis, I knew I was going to be Bob's advocate, without question, but being his caregiver?

I did know that in everyday conversation, the word caregiver had replaced the word caretaker, and I adopted the change in my speech so as not to appear old-fashioned. Caregiver, I kept repeating to myself. Not girlfriend, not lover, not partner, not wife. Caregiver.

As we drove home, Bob sat quietly and stared out the window. What a difference this day had made. I could see that he was tired from the trip and the meeting. We drove home in a silence that was unusual for us. I began to digest what Bob's illness, regardless of its name, and how it progressed, if it did, could mean for me. I had my first glimpse of this impending journey which cast me into a role with responsibilities I neither anticipated nor ever wanted.

CHAPTER 2

My Life Before Marriage

Bob and I were married on April 18, 1986, after having known each other for 15 years. Chalk up the delay to both of us having experienced unhappy first marriages. We found it difficult to summon the courage to make a legal commitment again.

Not until the morning of our wedding did we realize that the date we had chosen for our big day was the anniversary of the 1906 San Francisco earthquake. We were having breakfast in my condominium in the town of Alameda when we saw the headlines of the *San Francisco Chronicle* announcing the 80th anniversary of the quake. Bob said, "We've chosen the perfect date; only this time, the earth has stood still." We both laughed but didn't let the coincidence of the day frighten us about our decision to marry. We would drive to the town of Carmel in the Monterey Bay area for our very private marriage ceremony that afternoon. Just the two of us was what we had decided.

We planned to have lunch along the way. For sentimental reasons, we chose the historic La Casa Rosa restaurant in the Spanish mission town of San Juan Bautista. We had eaten there many times.

I was happy we made that choice. The day was warm, but the restaurant's patio was in the shade of laurel trees, which created an idyllic setting. We ordered our favorite — the Old California Casserole packed with cheese, tomato, and pepper flavors. It was romantic and the perfect beginning to our wedding weekend. After lunch, we drove to the Carmel Valley Lodge in time to check-in and change into our wedding outfits before the 5:00 marriage rite.

Through a couple of calls to the city offices of Carmel, Bob had arranged for a retired judge to perform the ceremony. The judge's wife would be our witness and their house, our wedding chapel. I liked the idea of the privacy and intimacy these arrangements would provide us. We would have to face our friends and family later if they were disappointed that we did not include them.

As we dressed — an off-white silk dress with delicate blue lines for me; a white dress shirt, striped silk tie, and navy blue suit for Bob — my mind wandered to the day we met. The year was 1970, and I had just turned 26. Bob was the branch manager of the sales office of Connecticut General Life Insurance Company (CGLIC) in Oakland, California.

Following an initial meeting with the office supervisor, Mr. Jacobs (as I was instructed to call him) would conduct the final interview and decide if I was to be the clerk-typist working part-time for him and part-time for the supervisor.

When I walked into his office, I was struck by his conservative appearance and formal approach as he introduced himself. For the previous two years, I had been teaching French and English in a high school in Southern California's Coachella Valley where the weather was hot most of the year. I was accustomed to seeing my male colleagues dressed informally in short-sleeve shirts without a tie or suit jacket. This business office would be quite a change for me.

I had recently moved to the San Francisco Bay Area to marry my first husband, Michael. We had met in Palm Desert, where I lived while teaching. When he relocated to Berkeley, we began to date long-distance and eventually, he proposed. I left the desert at the end of the school year to marry him.

Before I moved to Berkeley, I learned that the foreign language requirement for college admission had been withdrawn by the University of California, thus dramatically reducing the need for foreign language teachers. Since school districts in the Bay Area did not reply to my job application letters, I focused my job search on businesses.

However, employers seemed afraid to consider hiring me, given my prior employment as a teacher. They were direct about their concern that I would return to teaching as soon as a position was offered to me. I reduced my employment expectations to that of an entry-level administration position in any business and just hoped for an opportunity where I could get a start. I wanted this job at CGLIC—indeed, any employment with a chance to learn and progress.

The interview with the branch manager was notably different than the others I had that summer. From the introduction on, Mr. Jacobs treated me with a respect that I had learned not to count on in interviews. He seated himself behind a large rosewood table with matching credenza and pointed me to one of the two upholstered chairs in the middle of the room. He was a strawberry blond guy with a ruddy complexion and sturdy features. Good-looking, some would have said, but that was not my interest. He began by asking me about the languages I had studied in college. He seemed more interested in French and Italian than my administrative skills or my lack of previous business experience. I realized I was able to talk about my teaching experiences without fearing that I was setting myself up for rejection. I later learned that CGLIC, a New England company that was 100 years old, hired college graduates for many administrative positions.

CGLIC, or Mr. Jacobs specifically, hired me. I was eager to learn, not knowing where it might lead, but glad to have a start. I took on a variety of accounting and clerical tasks in my new job.

I found I liked office work and stayed at CGLIC for five years. One of my tasks was to type, copy, and mail the quarterly sales newsletter Mr. Jacobs wrote and illustrated. He began asking me my opinion about his writing, and I discovered we had a common interest in words and writing. It was fun to work together, and his sense of humor began to appear.

A promotion to staff secretary rewarded my work efforts, and sometime later, I was promoted to office supervisor, the most senior administrative position in the office. I supervised the clerical staff and reported directly to Mr. Jacobs. We worked well together, and I learned a lot about the insurance business from him. He seemed to be a natural teacher.

Sadly, less than two years after becoming the office supervisor, the primary job responsibilities of all office supervisors around the country were transferred to the corporate offices in Connecticut. This change signaled to me that it was time to find another job where I could grow and continue to learn. Having seen how sales agents' pay was directly connected to their performance, I also wanted a position where my contribution to the business could be more easily measured and appreciated.

I began the search for a new job with some enthusiasm as I was more confident than five years earlier, and my circumstances had changed. My marriage had been troubled from the beginning, and I had recently filed for divorce. I was prepared to work long hours and travel if needed. I moved to San Francisco and shared an apartment with a friend from college.

The next opportunity I found was in Oakland at the headquarters of PayLess Drug Stores of California and Hawaii. It meant a commute, but I liked the idea of being the administrative assistant for the clothing buyer. It looked like a great opportunity in the beginning, but a year into the job, I became frustrated that I would ever advance to be a buyer. Then a new manager was hired. He told me, in a bias typical of the times, that women buyers who traveled alone on buying trips to New York frequently developed reputations that he didn't think I would want. In essence, he blocked my promotion. I was disappointed and frustrated.

I didn't want to change jobs again so soon, and I worried over what I should do next. Then I remembered that Mr. Jacobs had offered to advise me about business situations when I left CG. We had met for lunch a couple of times, so I felt comfortable calling and asking for help.

I complained to Bob, no longer Mr. Jacobs to me, about my PayLess boss discouraging me from becoming a buyer. He casually said, "Why don't you find a job helping women advance in their careers? I think you'd really like that."

"Wow," I said. "What made you think of that?"

He shrugged his shoulders and gave me a look that said, "You'll figure it out." He had more confidence in me than I had in myself. I thanked him for his advice, but I couldn't imagine how to find a job like the one he described.

Surprisingly, a week later, I learned about a job opening within PayLess for a training and personnel administrator at the Northern Division office. I applied the next day, was interviewed, and within days was promoted to my first job in Human Resources (HR).

The primary responsibility required the recruitment of women and minorities for management training positions in the Division's 25 stores, most of which were in the East Bay. As it turned out, PayLess promoted me because they liked the fact that I had been a teacher, a supervisor, and had proven communication and organizational skills. Finally, my teaching experience was working for me instead of against me.

After I accepted the new job, I called Bob and thanked him for giving me the idea, but I did wonder if he had prescience. I gave him some of the details I had learned about the job so far. We agreed it was the perfect opportunity for me.

To meet the Division's recruitment goals, I would be traveling every week to interview candidates. It made sense for me to move to the East Bay, where I found a charming downstairs apartment in a large, older home. I also bought a new car and felt like I had settled into my new job and living alone.

Around the same time that I started my new HR job at PayLess, Bob left CGLIC to begin working for another insurance company. We began to see each other more often and enjoyed the times when we could get together. We discovered we had many interests in common. As time passed,

I began to wonder if I was falling in love with my former boss, mentor, and friend.

In 1980, another company bought the PayLess Drug Store chain. The new corporate owner laid off all employees in management positions. That layoff was to be the first of many, as companies I worked for that went through mergers and downsizing. Each new job carried more responsibility, and my expertise in HR management grew.

With each job change, my lack of a business degree was frequently a subject of discussion in the interviews. Potential employers would ask, "What do you know about HR with a degree in Romance Languages?" Frustrated by that bias, I began to explore MBA programs that I could pursue in the evening.

I told Bob I was thinking about graduate school. He was enthusiastic and encouraged me to apply. With his encouragement, I enrolled in the MBA program at Golden Gate University in San Francisco. The commitment meant five years of night school while I continued to work full-time. True to his word, Bob was always supportive and never complained when I said, "I'd love to go to the movies, but I have to study."

Some weekends, we spent time at Bob's apartment high above Oakland's Lake Merritt. It had an expansive, beautiful view of the lake from the living/dining room. For fun, we called it his "penthouse." One Sunday morning, I was studying at the dining room table while he read the newspaper, sitting next to the glass doors opening onto the balcony. I looked up to see him relaxed with the view of the lake behind him.

I said, for no reason, "Do you love me?"

He quickly responded, "It's easier than not to."

"What?" I asked, not knowing if I had heard him correctly. Once I saw his face, I knew he was teasing. Then we both burst out laughing. It was difficult to concentrate again on my studies, but it was so typical of the kind of fun we could have, even when I had to study.

After the last night of my final class in graduate school in December 1985, I walked out of the building on Mission Street in San Francisco at 10:00 p.m. To my surprise, Bob was waiting for me. I didn't need a ride home and immediately wondered what he was doing there. Then I saw he was holding a dozen red roses and a bottle of champagne.

"Congratulations! You made it, Cher," he declared with a big smile. The unexpected recognition was so great, I started to cry. He held me until I could regain my composure.

This wonderful man, and he alone, had seen me through this lengthy endeavor to obtain an MBA. I knew how proud of me he was—even more than my family. By now, I felt that Bob and I had become partners, and we could face whatever the future might bring.

Some months after graduation, my friend Elizabeth, who had moved to the Napa Valley, called me. She was a friend from my days at PayLess. I visited her in Napa from time to time, and the beauty and tranquility of the Valley appealed to me. Elizabeth worked at Napa Valley Bank, but I was not expecting the question that she asked, "Would you be interested in applying for the Vice President of Human Resources at the bank?" I was surprised and thrilled at this unexpected opportunity. It meant I would be responsible for the bank's HR department and a big step up for me.

The decision to apply for the job was easy. Furthermore, I had thought often about how I might like to live in the

Napa Valley. I told Bob about the opportunity and was pleased that he thought the Napa Valley would be an excellent place for him to retire sometime in the future.

As for our age difference, it had never seemed a problem to us, but would it be as the years passed? He thought he might be able to ask for a job transfer to a location closer to Napa. The idea of Bob commuting some 50 miles each way made me think about his age and the demands of a long drive twice a day.

And what about our future? By now, we both were divorced and free to live wherever we might choose. I had no children; Bob had three adult children — Lisa, Cindy, and Peter — all living in different parts of the country.

Yes, we had talked about marriage, but my job change put the topic front and center. There were practical considerations too. Both of us owned homes in the Bay Area, so there were several financial issues to consider and, most importantly, our fears about committing to marriage again. Meanwhile, we were both honest with ourselves that a community bank in an agricultural area might be conservative enough to disapprove of a couple living together without being married.

"I don't want my living arrangement to influence how the bank's executives view me," I told him.

He nodded in agreement and then asked, "Are you sure you want to get involved with a bank?" I knew he had worked in banking and thought banks had very political environments.

I told him I was not worried about a community bank. I reminded him that I had already seen the organizational challenges in many types of businesses, in addition to a recent contract position I had held at the San Francisco Federal

Home Loan Bank. I was not concerned about the banking business as much as leaving the Bay Area urban lifestyle and moving to a small town, which I had happily left when I went to college.

I did not change my mind, although I thought the bank had. It took them a long time to finalize their decision about hiring me after I had driven to the Napa Valley for three separate interviews. They finally offered me the position with a start date of May 1, some six weeks away. I accepted.

The work decision finalized, our living arrangement still needed to be decided. One evening at dinner at a small café we frequented, I said, "I think we've talked about this for some time. Let's take the leap and get married."

Bob nodded his head with a big smile on his face and reached across the table to hold my hand. "You're so right. And I have been thinking more and more about retirement. Getting married and moving to the Napa Valley sounds perfect."

The evening ended with our deciding we needed to talk about the logistical details since my start date at the bank was not far away. It was a big step for both of us. And, finally, joyfully, we took it. I arrived on my first day of work in the Napa Valley, a newly married woman.

CHAPTER 3

The Pursuit of a Diagnosis

The first seven years of our marriage were almost idyllic. We loved living in the Napa Valley, especially since Bob retired not long after our move there. For the first time, he was able to pursue his interests in volunteering. After extensive training, Bob became a lay counselor at the Community Counseling Center, an advocate for foster children at CASA (Court Appointed Special Advocates), and a friendly visitor to recently released patients from the local hospital. He enjoyed classes in art and wine at the local community college. He also joined the Senior Center's choir, which performed at retirement facilities in the Napa Valley. I worked long hours at my job in banking and loved both the work and my colleagues. We splurged too, having our house remodeled and traveling to Europe. Life was predictable and enjoyable.

Then in 1993, Napa Valley Bank was sold to a large regional bank. I saw the sale as a chance to make a leap that Bob and I had talked about at length; I wanted to have my own business as a one-person human resources consultant. I knew there were many small businesses in the North Bay that needed human resources expertise from time to time but were too small to have an HR expert on staff. Those businesses were ready-made clients for me.

Finally, we decided to give the idea a year and see if I could make a go of it. Although we would need to adjust to a reduction in pay at the beginning and the loss of my benefits package, the significant advantages would mean being my own boss and working from my home office.

My one-year trial as Cheri J. Bailly-Jacobs, Human Resources Consultant, became eight years, at which time our lives changed dramatically.

After a childhood of intermittent and undiagnosed stomachaches, Bob's stomach problems reappeared with some regularity in 2000. Following several trips to the emergency room and more frequent pain that doubled him over, in the early summer of 2001, he was diagnosed with a twisted colon. It required emergency surgery. That meant almost a week in the hospital, then a colostomy for three months, and follow-up surgery to undo the colostomy with another week in the hospital. When the second surgery was successful, the surgeon assured us that the problem would not reoccur. It did not. By then, however, my magical thinking about Bob's health and our future was shaken.

During his stays in the hospital, some 15 miles away, I continued with my regular work schedule, fitting in trips to visit him at least once a day, and feeling in a daze most of the time. In Bob's early retirement, while I concentrated on my consulting work, I had counted on him to take care of the many responsibilities of running our household and managing our finances.

Then came a shocker. One afternoon while Bob was in the hospital, I took a minute to check some papers on his desk. There I saw a cancellation letter from our auto insurance carrier. I immediately called the insurance company and made arrangements to reinstate the policy that day.

When Bob came home from the hospital, I immediately asked him about it. "Did you pay the car insurance bill before your surgery?"

"Oh, yeah, some time ago, I think," he responded. His answer didn't ring true. By now, I had gone through the checkbook for household expenses, and there was no check for the insurance.

When I questioned him more closely, he just looked at me.

I expected a reaction showing his surprise like, "Oh, my God, how could that be?" Instead, he said, "But we have insurance, right?" and began to shuffle through papers on the desk as if the conversation were over.

I decided to reassure him I had made arrangements for payment and the policy had been reinstated.

Finally, he said, "Okay, then we're all set."

I still waited for him to scratch his head as he sometimes did and try to figure out what had happened. Instead, he said, "I think I'll lie down. All of a sudden, I feel tired."

The missed insurance payment was a clue, but one I did not recognize at the time.

I had taken on the duties of president of the Napa Chamber of Commerce that year, a time-consuming volunteer job I fit in between writing proposals, doing projects, and responding to clients' crisis calls. ("We think one of our employees is stealing from us. Can you meet with us this afternoon?") Sometimes I felt as if I were floating from one world to the next in a kind of fog. I remember one day visiting Bob in the hospital in the morning, leaving early enough to travel back to Napa to lead the monthly

Chamber Board of Directors' meeting, and somewhere in between checking my voice mail for client calls.

For the first time, married life felt out of control without having Bob to count on.

I thought I had married the healthiest 58-year-old man on the planet. When I made the traditional promises at our marriage ceremony, I was confident I could live by all the vows the judge asked me to repeat. The words "in sickness and in health" did not make me hesitate in the slightest. I would have been shocked, however, if he had added, "and act as lifetime caregiver for your spouse if he gets any form of dementia."

Although I was 17 years younger than Bob, he seemed my age physically and took excellent care of himself. He loved to eat fruits and vegetables. Salty or sweet snacks never tempted him, and generally, he had what we now call a "heart-healthy diet." He was disciplined about exercise: jogging or riding his bike at least three times a week, doing stretching exercises after a workout, and playing tennis most Saturdays. I used to tell him, "You'll outlive me, I'm sure."

However, after Bob's colon problems were resolved and he was back home, he began to struggle with depression. That fall, on his own, he arranged to see a psychiatrist, who prescribed Prozac. At the next couple of visits, when Bob told him he wasn't feeling better, the doctor increased the dosage.

In January of 2002, just days after Bob's doctor prescribed him the most recent Prozac increase, Bob and I took our postponed vacation when my year with the Chamber of Commerce had ended. We decided on a road trip to one of our favorite short vacation spots, Palm Springs, then on to Tucson, Arizona, for a more extended stay.

On the first leg of the drive, Bob was not his usual positive self. He used to love road trips, but I hadn't seen much enthusiasm this time. I told myself this was part of his recovery from surgery, as well as an intermittent tooth pain that had bothered him for a few weeks. And I told myself, perhaps the increased dosage of the Prozac had not yet kicked in. In case the tooth pain became worse, I packed some leftover Vicodin and tried to think positively.

Then one evening in Palm Springs, Bob announced he didn't want to drive back to the hotel from the restaurant, as he was unable to figure out where we were in the dark. We had visited Palm Springs many times and always stayed at the same hotel. I was surprised by his reluctance, so I asked him why. He said, "I don't know which way the streets run, and I don't think I can find the hotel." I didn't pursue his explanation and decided to think about it later. I wanted to enjoy our trip and give my brain a real break from any problem-solving.

By the time we had been in Arizona a couple of days, the tooth pain resurfaced. Bob was miserable. I gave him Vicodin, but the pain was still bothersome. Also, he seemed to become more confused and withdrawn. I reasoned that the Vicodin (and maybe the increased dosage of Prozac) were the culprits. We cut the trip short and headed for home.

During the return trip, I told Bob I'd like to accompany him to his next appointment with the psychiatrist. I was beginning to worry about his mental abilities and wanted to make the doctor aware of my concerns. I also was trying to convince myself there was nothing wrong with Bob that stopping the drugs couldn't fix.

When we met with his psychiatrist the following week, his response to my concerns was, "If the cure is worse than the disease, we stop the cure." He gave us instructions on slowly reducing Bob's Prozac. Although the appointment was short, I left the doctor's office with optimism that perhaps we had found the culprit.

But after the Prozac was out of Bob's system, there was no discernible change in his mood. His less than typically sunny attitude concerned me, but his behavior began to worry me more. I began to imagine that my quick acceptance of the psychiatrist's answer to Bob's problems was actually my denial.

As Bob and I worked on our tax preparation in early 2002, I noticed he was having difficulty completing his part of our accountant's annual questionnaire. When we sat down at the breakfast table to go over medical expenses, he became confused and agitated, thumbing through the papers almost in a panic. He said, "We have to stop. I need to go over these numbers by myself. Something isn't right here."

I had heard this complaint from him twice before when we started the medical expenses part of the questionnaire. This time I said, "Bob, you've gone over these totals a couple of times now. We're running out of time. Let's enter the numbers you have. I'm sure they're fine." In frustration, he agreed.

By now, I had also seen Bob struggle with his calendar. He had lived by a daily planner for years, yet now was showing up late for haircuts, getting into difficulties with his chorus leader for his lateness, and seemed confused way too often. I'd thought of all the things that could be wrong with him; the word Alzheimer's was something I did not allow myself to consider.

I did recall that Bob's brother, eight years older, had been struggling with some memory problems. He had told us that the problem was diagnosed as small strokes. I focused on that as a possibility and imagined a brain tumor as well. I kept my thoughts to myself, hoping something else might surface to explain his problems.

By chance, I read an article in an AARP magazine about Aricept, a medicine for Alzheimer's disease. Upon learning it was only useful during the early part of the disease, I was spurred to action and decided to approach Bob about seeing his doctor for a checkup.

One night after dinner, I introduced my concern. I said, "I want to ask a favor of you. It's because there is such an age difference between us; I need to talk to you about something." I thought that mentioning our age difference would somehow reinforce the reasonableness of my request. I carefully said, "I recently read about a drug for Alzheimer's. It's only prescribed during the early part of the disease." I paused to watch his reaction. Although this was the first time I used the word "Alzheimer's" with him, he seemed fine, so I proceeded. "I've noticed some problems recently, like with the taxes. I'm a bit concerned. Would you be willing to see your doctor and be tested for Alzheimer's?"

"Sure," he quickly said with a smile. To my surprise, he didn't seem upset at all.

I was so relieved, I stood up and gave him a big hug and said, "Oh, thank you. That's great."

We agreed to start with his primary care physician at Kaiser Permanente. We were both members of a Kaiser health plan, which made it easy for each of us to be in touch with the other's health situation. Our doctor knew Bob to be a healthy 74-year-old. She was also my doctor, so I felt confident she would work openly with the two of us. I also knew that my usual mode of worry, which often verged on pessimism, was now best hidden.

I felt fortunate he was cooperative. I learned later that not all people with early signs of memory challenges are willing to acknowledge that there might be a problem. I was told many times how lucky I was that Bob was so willing to investigate this potential health problem.

At the first appointment, she gave Bob a brief exam, checked his blood pressure, listened to his heart, and asked questions about the kinds of memory problems he was having. She said the next step would be a blood test. Ordering lab work seemed standard procedure to me. I was relieved she didn't have a dementia diagnosis at the ready, nor say the words, "Well, Bob is getting older."

A week later, when we met with his doctor to review the blood panel results, she went through the items one by one, "Your B-12 level is fine. Sometimes when there isn't enough B-12 in the system, it can cause memory problems." Bob and I smiled at each other, knowing how disciplined he was about diet and exercise.

Then she calmly said, "The blood test also confirms that you don't have syphilis." I had to run that sentence through my head a couple of times to assure myself that she said, "...*do not* have syphilis." The one thing I did not expect to hear at this appointment was a reference to venereal disease. Bob and I had been married for a long time; a diagnosis of that kind would have shattered my trust and our relationship. It took me a few minutes to recover from hearing the word syphilis applied to Bob.

Finally, one of us said, "Well, that's a relief."

The doctor did not explain why she felt she needed to tell us of the non-existence of such a disease. Either she was being thorough or thought we needed good news. We did, but not that.

She finished the meeting by saying, "Let's get you a CT scan, and I'll make a referral to a neurologist who will review the results with you." The fact that she was ordering another test and passing us on to a specialist made me feel hopeful but anxious. Bob had not received a clean bill of health yet—something I was unconsciously counting on every day—and we still knew nothing about his brain.

I did remind myself that a referral to a specialist was standard procedure at Kaiser. You start with the primary care physician, then move on to specialists when the primary care physician determines it necessary.

Two weeks later, we drove to a Kaiser Medical Center, in a town nearby, to see a neurologist. I was nervous but tried not to look it, as I showed Bob's membership card and driver's license to the female receptionist at the Neurology Department. Bob was friendly, making conversation with her, and acting as if he were looking forward to the appointment. In short, he was his usual optimistic self, while my pessimism made me afraid of hearing the worst.

Shown to a room to wait for the doctor, Bob jumped up on the exam table as if he were a frequent patient who knew his way around. Then he pointed at the doctor's diplomas on the wall and said, "This is the same neurologist I saw a couple of years ago." He went on to explain the neurologist had examined him following a minor car accident. No wonder Bob was so relaxed; he was in familiar territory.

When the doctor walked through the door, his white coat neatly buttoned, he was all business. He put a file on the desk, sat down, but didn't greet us in any way. There was no "Hello" or "How are you?" Bob broke the silence playfully and with a smile asked, "Are you going to give me that same test you gave me last time?"

The doctor, never looking at Bob, said, "I don't know. Based on the way your CT scan looks, I'm surprised you haven't peed on my exam table and were able to walk in here."

I didn't know what to do. The doctor clearly meant to take charge of the meeting. He must not have remembered or cared that he had seen Bob before. I guessed Bob's attempt at humor about the test must have irritated him. He continued to look down at his file. Bob and I sat in silence. If I had been able to think of a question, I might have asked it, but the whole meeting was going in an unexpected direction. I could not understand the doctor's insolence.

Finally, he walked over to the exam table and gave Bob what I considered to be a cursory neurological exam, taking no more than ten minutes. He tested Bob's reactions to taps on his joints with a small rubber hammer and looked in his eyes with a flashlight. With no explanation, he asked Bob a series of questions I later learned were part of a test called the Mini-Mental Status Examination, a quick way to assess memory and cognitive functions.

"Do you know what city you are in? Who is the President of the United States? I'm going to give you three words and later I'll ask you to recall them for me."

Oh no, I thought. This might not be so easy, but Bob was able to recall the words at the appropriate time.

Lastly, the doctor said, "Count backward by 7's from 100."

Without hesitation, Bob answered, "100, 93, 86, (then a small pause), 79, 72."

At that point, the doctor interrupted him. "That's enough."

I remembered that Bob, always a good test taker in school, did quite well on everything. The doctor said nothing more. With no discussion or comment on Bob's test score, he said, "Come across the hall into my office. I want to show you Bob's CT scan."

We followed him like obedient children. He turned the lights on a wall screen, and the scan of Bob's brain appeared. He said, "The concern is that there are so many parts of Bob's brain that show up black."

It was the first time I had seen a brain scan. I could see black areas, but that didn't help me understand what was going on. I could see the shape of his brain but couldn't make out anything else except areas of black alongside areas of gray. My mind was racing with the possibilities of what the scan meant, as I waited for more information. The doctor offered nothing.

Bob was quiet as he continued to stare at the screen. I wondered if he had any idea what the scan represented.

I felt a lump in my throat and feared I would start to cry if I asked a question, but eventually managed to ask, "What does that mean?"

"It means those black areas are water. Nature abhors a vacuum. As the cells have disappeared, water has replaced them." End of explanation.

He walked behind his desk and sat down. We continued to stand. "I'll write you a prescription for Aricept." He offered no explanation about the medication. I assumed he thought we knew what it was for. He handed it to Bob and stood up, indicating the appointment was over.

I was unable to ask anything else. I didn't want to talk about Alzheimer's with this aloof doctor, so we learned precious little about Bob's condition or what to do next. I didn't ask for a diagnosis but wish I had. I also didn't ask for another appointment. I felt dismissed.

Looking back on that awful day, I think my unexpressed anger paralyzed me. We had never been treated like this at Kaiser before. And my fear that the news was not good also kept me silent. Even though I knew that Aricept was for the early stages of Alzheimer's, I couldn't process the possibility that Bob had the disease. I also knew that Bob wasn't familiar with drug names, so he had not connected the name Aricept with Alzheimer's.

As we exited the building, I took Bob's hand, more for my reassurance than his, and we walked in silence to the parking lot. When we drove away and started to talk, surprisingly, we were both a bit giddy. I think we were relieved that the appointment was over. We drove home smiling and laughing at what a jerk the doctor had been. Humor had often been a way for us to survive tough times, and that is what we naturally turned to. Although I didn't say anything to Bob about the non-diagnosis, I was temporarily comforted by the fact that, apparently, no brain tumor was present in the CT scan. The whole tone of the appointment, not to mention the lack of information, was health care almost at its worst.

After such a disappointing neurology appointment, we decided not to go back to our primary care doctor. She had done her job and sent us to an appropriate specialist. Further help from her would probably not be forthcoming.

Then, entirely on his own, Bob telephoned the Alzheimer's Association. I don't know how he decided to do this, how he got the number, or what his thinking was. This kind of unanticipated take-charge behavior is one aspect of memory loss that I would learn is crazy-making for the caregiver. Just when you think someone can't do a task, all of a sudden he's done it. I asked, "How did you know to call them?"

He didn't have an explanation, but he was enthusiastic about the information he had received and couldn't wait to tell me. "The Alzheimer's Association told me to call a research center at the University of California at Davis." Later we were to learn that there were ten such Alzheimer's Research Centers located in university medical centers throughout California. In addition to conducting research, these centers help those with Alzheimer's disease by providing comprehensive assessments of individuals with memory problems. At the time Bob called them, they were eager to schedule assessments without a referral or a fee. It felt like our luck was beginning to change.

Although we knew very little about what the assessment might include, Bob and I were both eager to talk to research professionals who might give us more information than we'd been able to gather from our two previous doctor visits.

Bob made the call to arrange an appointment which would be at the Veteran's Hospital in the town of Martinez, 40 miles south of Napa. The assessment was scheduled for

August, a couple of months away. Only after his call did it dawn on us that we had committed to a three-week vacation that month to visit family in Oregon, Washington, and New Jersey. Bob's biggest pleasure in life was to travel; I didn't want to take that away when he could still enjoy it. Neither of us wanted to cancel the trip so I called and rescheduled the appointment.

I called the Center again and explained to them that Bob had been prescribed Aricept by a doctor at Kaiser. I asked if a delay in starting the Aricept would be a problem. They assured me it would be all right, and they would prefer that he not start the medication because they wanted to conduct their tests without the Aricept in his system. It never occurred to me that they might prescribe something else, or maybe nothing at all.

The vacation went well, with no changes in Bob's abilities that I could notice. After our return, the day of our appointment at the Alzheimer's Disease Center finally arrived. I had explicit driving directions, but since it was somewhere in a large Veterans' Administration complex, in our usual mode of punctuality, we left early to be sure to be on time. At the Center, the office staff warmly greeted us, a direct contrast to the neurologist. The receptionist gave us a few forms to complete, and I assured Bob I would fill out the paperwork. So far, so good.

When it was time for Bob's testing, a research psychologist came to the waiting area and introduced herself. She explained the testing process would take about three hours and would consist of pencil and paper tests, a brief medical exam, and interviews by a neuropsychologist, a neurologist, a psychologist, and the research team nurse practitioner. I was to be interviewed as well, which was a welcome surprise. I wanted to tell the researchers what I had observed in Bob's behavior and give them some examples of the memory problems he experienced.

When Bob was taken away for testing, I turned to some consulting work I had brought with me. When, hours later, I was invited into a room to meet with the nurse practitioner, she started the interview by asking me, "How are you doing as Bob's caregiver?"

Neither our primary care doctor nor the neurologist had asked me how I was doing. I felt tears come to my eyes, and it took me a few minutes before I could regain my composure. Only then did I realize that for the past year, his needs required more from me than I had wanted to acknowledge. I began to grasp how concerned I had been for both Bob and me.

The nurse was so gentle and reassuring that in a few minutes, I was able to carry on a conversation. We went through several questions about what I had observed and experienced with Bob since noticing the memory problems. I felt my opinions and ideas were essential to the assessment. Being included made me feel better about everything.

After the nurse finished with her questions, she told me to stay in that room because the neuropsychologist wanted to interview me too. His interview was shorter than hers but involved similar questions. When he completed his questionnaire, he asked if I had any questions. I surprised myself by asking, "What about drinking? Bob likes wine with dinner every night. Can he continue to do that?"

There was a pause, and then he said, "If I had something going on with my central nervous system, I wouldn't use alcohol anymore." I thanked him for his frankness and saved his advice so I could carefully pass it on to Bob at the right time.

Back in the waiting room, I found Bob with the nurse. She explained we were finished and would receive a call about setting a conference date to share the findings. We were also encouraged to include family members in the meeting. We were graciously thanked for our participation in the research and left to find ourselves a place for lunch.

When we left the office, Bob and I were both cheerful and pleased at how things had gone, different than the nervous laughs we experienced after seeing the Kaiser neurologist. He was exhausted, though. I was learning he had much less energy than in earlier times. Again, I reached for his hand. I felt we were partners in whatever was to come.

The family conference at the Center later that month included all the interviewers on the research team and Bob and me. Through the Center's assistance, Bob's adult children were able to participate via conference call. I had mentioned to all three of them that Bob was experiencing some memory problems, so the arrangement of the call was not a shock to them. It was a relief that they would hear the researchers' findings on the phone and not from my later recall of the meeting.

The conclusions, carefully and cautiously explained by each researcher, were that Bob had Mild Cognitive Impairment which they referred to as MCI. And, the neurologist said, "MCI could advance to Alzheimer's disease." Could, I noted to myself. Not would.

But, they added, because this diagnosis was new and limited data was available about progression to Alzheimer's, there was no way of telling if Alzheimer's would occur in Bob's case. I looked at Bob for a reaction, but he seemed focused on only taking in everything the research team said.

The neurologist also explained that Aricept might postpone future symptoms, and it was imperative to be consistent in taking it. "Some patients begin to feel better after taking Aricept and then stop taking it," she warned. She added if Bob were to stop taking the medication, restarting it might not help his condition.

The staff also gave us some information about resources—mostly the names of agencies that offered at-home care to provide respite for caregivers. Most were not near us, but the listings did give me an idea of what I should begin to research in our area.

Bob and I now had a diagnosis and some information about Aricept. He could start taking the medication. On the way home, we talked about how this was about the best outcome we could have hoped for at this point. We could begin to plan the next phase of our lives. The MCI diagnosis seemed so much less dramatic than my worst fears; it gave us some hope and optimism. We would need both.

Part Two

Learning to Live with the Early Stages

CHAPTER 4

Who to Tell?

After the few weeks Bob and I needed to absorb the news of the MCI diagnosis, another question began to surface for me: Who would, or should, we tell and how much should we say? Bob's adult children already knew about his memory problems, as they had been a part of the family phone conference at UC Davis. I had told my mother, brother, and sister we were searching for a diagnosis, but I asked them not to mention it to others until we were more confident about what was going on. My father had suffered from vascular dementia, and my mother knew only too well the possible future we were facing. I reasoned there was no need to worry any of them until necessary. And Bob looked like a healthy guy, still driving the car, riding his bike, singing in the community chorus, and enjoying his retirement.

Then I recalled an experience that happened not long after we had moved into our new home. A woman who lived across the street had attached a handwritten note to our front door. I didn't know her well. We had waved to each other as we pulled our cars out of the driveway but rarely chatted about neighborhood happenings. Her note was short and to the point. If her husband was found wandering around the cul-de-sac, we were asked to notify her as soon as possible. The note explained that he was unable to speak and, therefore, might be in some distress in her absence. I was struck at the time how scary this would be for both of them if neighbors did not know about the man's condition.

With a future image of Bob wandering around our neighborhood, I decided to talk with him first about whom he wanted to tell about his memory loss and when. One evening in the kitchen, after a good meal of grilled salmon and brown rice (one of his favorites), I started by telling him I thought we needed to discuss what he wanted to share with others about his health condition. He nodded and waited for me to go on.

I said, "As you know, your kids already know about the MCI diagnosis, and I have told my mom, brother, and sister we are concerned about your memory, but nobody else knows anything. Do you feel okay telling others, including some of the neighbors and friends?"

He again nodded, "Yes."

I waited until he was ready to speak and realized I was still adjusting to the extra time it took for him to answer questions. Lately, he limited his comments until he knew where I was headed.

Finally, he said, "I'm fine with people knowing I have memory problems. I don't know about going into all the details."

I replied, "Okay, I think we agree." I wanted to repeat what I thought the agreement was, to make sure I didn't only hear what I wanted. "I'd like us to tell people about your memory when we feel it is appropriate. For example, I'd like to tell the neighbors right away."

Bob said, "I think that would be good too."

I suggested I do the communicating. As soon as I offered that, I could see him relax. I felt a considerable relief, knowing we had the same attitude about not creating a family secret. This delicate conversation ended in a big hug. I still felt so safe in his arms, even though I knew other responsibilities were coming my way. I wasn't sure I was ready for all of them, but carefully getting the word out about Bob's memory would be a significant first step.

Before I started to tell any neighbor Bob's story, I had it fairly well planned. My announcement would be short and to the point with little or no references to medical words: "Bob has been diagnosed with early-stage memory loss, but we don't know if it will progress to Alzheimer's disease. We want to be open about it. Some people seem to feel a lot of shame about Alzheimer's; we don't want to be a part of that. We both want you to know that if you ever see Bob looking lost or confused, you'll have a clue as to what might be happening with him."

I started my careful recital with our neighbor Teresa. Her kids always took care of our cats when we went on vacation, and we had developed an easy friendship with the family. Teresa's response was just what I hoped for. She listened carefully and quickly offered to be of help if I needed something. It was a good start; the other neighbors were also caring and showed concern about Bob. I felt comforted that "telling" was the right thing to do.

Telling my clients was a bit more complicated. I rarely shared personal information with clients and did not want them to insert themselves into Bob's health situation by offering suggestions or recommendations for his care. Finally, I decided I needed to be open with them as well, so they wouldn't wonder why I wasn't as available as before. Everyone was empathetic and helpful. They reassured me they understood the pressures I was under and that whenever I needed to change an appointment, just let them know. Again, disclosure was another significant relief.

With many of our friends or acquaintances, however, I rarely got past the first sentence. They frequently interrupted me to say, "Oh, I know what you mean. I lose my keys all the time." Or they would tell their own story about their grandmother who had Alzheimer's. I ended up being the listener. In those circumstances, I felt dismissed and had to work hard not to be angry. I was also disappointed they did not even acknowledge Bob's and my situation. How could anyone expect me to focus on their story when I was struggling with the new realities of Bob's health and what the future held for both of us?

Gradually, I was able to understand their responses were a function of being uncomfortable with hearing the news about Bob and perhaps their fears about the disease. While I missed feeling the support I was hoping for, it confirmed my instincts that we needed to get memory loss and its devastating effects on families out in the open. In the absence of a medical breakthrough, talking about memory loss, it seemed to me, was the best that we as individuals could do.

In time, I grew more selective regarding whom I spoke to about Bob's situation. And it became easier to speak the words once I grew accustomed to responses that ranged from total silence to an abrupt change of subject. I was especially thankful for some friends who did say, "I'm so sorry. Is there anything that I can do?" I never had a suggestion that I could think of at the moment. I later realized that I could have said, "We would love a pot of soup when you have some free time." Most people would have been relieved to have a way to help. As Bob's disease progressed, our decision not to keep it a secret became even more essential.

CHAPTER 5

Alarmed by Problems with Easy Tasks

On most days during the next couple of years, Bob drove into town—downtown Napa is located about four miles from our home—to run errands to places familiar to him. These forays were helpful to me, of course, but when he was late returning home, I became distressed and usually thought the worst. Did he have an accident? Had he gotten lost? Was he wandering around a shopping center not knowing where he was? Although nothing like this had ever happened, I knew that his memory was getting worse, and I had no idea what symptoms might appear when.

I learned to keep the errands list to a small number, but sometimes, I got overly ambitious. One afternoon, I put four stops on Bob's "To Do" list: return books to the library; buy a chicken at Vallerga's, a grocery store; buy a bottle of aspirin at the pharmacy; take sweaters to the cleaners. As we stood at the kitchen island and went over the list, I began to notice how muddled he seemed. He was dressed and ready to leave but stared at the paper as if in a daze. My explanation or the tasks themselves were causing him confusion.

Interrupting my instructions, I said, "It's okay, Bob. I'll just make a list with the two things I really need to have done today." He seemed to relax and pay more attention as I turned the piece of paper over with a dramatic gesture, partly out of frustration and also hoping that the visual of a new list on the other side would stay in his mind. I then rewrote two tasks and repeated the words out loud as I wrote them. "Take the books to the library, and buy a whole chicken at the grocery store, okay? Now, where do you want to keep the list? In your shirt pocket? Okay, there. You're all set." I realized I had sped up the usual explanation because I was out of patience. I needed Bob to head out and let me get back to my consulting work in my office down the hall.

"No problem, babe. I'm on my way," he said. Sometimes I think he was out of patience with me too. Off he went.

I returned to my work and didn't check the clock until I looked out the French doors in my office and noticed it was getting dark. Reassuring myself that Bob would be back momentarily, I resumed finishing plans for my meeting the next day.

When I heard the garage door open and looked at my watch, I was surprised to see that two hours had passed since I saw darkness beginning. Bob had been gone for over three hours. Grateful he was home and presumably safe, I quickly walked through the house to greet him in the kitchen.

He looked embarrassed and frustrated but volunteered what had happened. "I did fine at the library, except I tried to find some videos and couldn't, so then I looked for some CDs."

He presented me with six CDs, some of which he wasn't sure why he had chosen. "Then, I got the chicken and decided to go to Walmart to get the aspirin you wanted."

Aspirin? I said to myself. No, that was only on the original list.

He continued, "So when I went to Walmart, I took the chicken in with me." In our Walmart, no groceries or meats were available, so I imagined how he might have looked to other shoppers, pushing a shopping cart around the store containing a fresh chicken in a transparent plastic bag. "Nobody said anything when I checked out." He laughed at this, and I wanted to laugh as well but was too upset to see the humor.

"Bob, where's the list with just the two errands on it?"

"I don't know," he said. I pointed to his shirt pocket. The look of disbelief on his face told me he'd forgotten he even had a list. He then announced that he had considered going to get gas in the car but changed his mind because he wondered if it might be getting late. He was proud of how he had made that decision and thought I would be pleased too.

Seeing his pride helped me hide my feelings, struggling as I was with a combination of frustration and sadness. Bob enjoyed going to town; it not only broke up his day, he liked the fact that doing some errands provided assistance to me, and he still loved to drive. The last thing I wanted was to make him feel incapable and useless. Now I couldn't deny the fact that he was losing some of his ability to do everyday tasks, including remembering to read a list in his pocket.

"Let's get dinner going," I said. Talking about his lateness and confusion would not be beneficial to either of us at that point. And I did not want to think about what this day might mean about the future. I would try to think about that later.

CHAPTER 6

Unexpected Distress

I t was almost noon when I drove around the corner into our cul-de-sac and simultaneously clicked the garage door opener on the windshield visor. I was running a little late returning from my morning client appointment, but I tried not to drive faster than the neighborhood speed limit. There was just enough time to make myself a quick lunch, then head out to my next appointment, among other obligations I needed to meet before the end of the day.

When I opened the door from the garage into the kitchen, I saw Bob bent over the counter, holding his handkerchief to his face and crying almost uncontrollably.

"What's happened? Are you all right?" I asked as I rushed to him. He was facing two pieces of mismatched bread that I reasoned was supposed to be a sandwich.

Bob shook his head no. Immediately, I went into fix-it mode. I guided him to sit at the kitchen table, trying to reassure him by saying, "Let me get you an apple." Off to the refrigerator, I went to find a crisp apple that would somehow make everything okay. Then I realized he was still crying. My hurried soothing had done little to reassure him.

Could there be a problem with his lunch? Most days, I was home to make it with him, but some days, he was more on his own. I did not think he was in real trouble, but he couldn't stop crying to tell me what was wrong.

I went back to the table and bent down to hold him while he cried, knowing by now that sometimes his crying had a long life. And I also knew by now that trying to stop the crying by pushing food in front of him wouldn't make any pain—physical or emotional—go away.

As I held him, the chronology of what had happened came out in short, interrupted phrases. "I had trouble. Making the pieces of bread. Line up right." He held his breath and tried not to cry at what I thought he must have realized: He could no longer make a sandwich in what he considered the right way, that is, squared off.

"Then, when I tried to eat the sandwich, I choked on the lettuce." Bob liked lettuce with most sandwiches, but choking was new and probably scary for him. He took out his handkerchief and blew his nose slightly, folding his cloth handkerchief into a small ball, a long-time habit, before replacing it in his pants' pocket. "It really scared me."

While I tried to comfort him and not think about my upcoming client appointment, I recognized a familiar truth: As soon as I believe that I've seen most of what triggers confusion and frustration in Bob's troubled mind, I learn something new. But I was increasingly in a quandary. I'd been told over and over that routine is so vital in dealing with dementia-related symptoms. But Bob always liked new things, loved to travel, and still seemed open to trying almost anything. Was all of that gone already, just two years since his diagnosis? That day, I could hardly think about such a significant issue, so I moved on to practical problem-solving and my typical solution of "Let's make a plan."

I waited a bit more until he seemed calm. "When I'm not home, I'll write out the lunch menu on one of the blank index cards. I'll go over it with you and leave the card on the island. How does that sound?" He nodded as he tried again to eat the sandwich. Thinking of writing out a daily menu would mean one more task to add to my duties, and I suddenly felt annoyed. I was aware of the pressure of time, and I needed to eat and be on my way.

I returned to the refrigerator finally to make myself lunch and decided to leave Bob with his sandwich. I often made the mistake of talking too much when he was struggling with something. As I ate, I watched him out of the corner of my eye. He seemed to be settled down and was eating without difficulty.

A few minutes later, I said, "I'm off to my next meeting, sweetie. I'll be home in a couple of hours." I knew I had to hit the road for my afternoon appointment in order to be on time. "Maybe we can go for a walk then."

He nodded in agreement but didn't look up at me. I kissed him on the cheek and headed for the garage.

I wanted to get out of the house and go back to my world of work. There were always challenges in my business, but I could count on certain assumptions that didn't change every time I turned around. And sandwiches were not something I would have to worry about.

CHAPTER 7

My Absence Creates Problems

I had been teaching business management classes at Santa Rosa Junior College in neighboring Sonoma County since 1998. On my teaching days, I usually left home at 6:30 a.m. on Saturday and returned twelve hours later. It was a long day for me, but the teaching was challenging and different from consulting. I also thought it might be a way eventually to ease into retirement.

Before the time of such long days, I was usually gone from home not more than three hours, mostly to meet with a client. On such occasions, Bob stayed at home by himself. The twelve-hour teaching day, however, created new challenges for both of us. I would fix his lunch and place the sandwich in the refrigerator with a note on it so he could easily find it. I printed a couple of suggestions on a large index card, listing what he might do while I was gone (look at his books of nature photos or watch his favorite Broadway musicals DVD). I always included my contact information at the college. I left the card on the island in the kitchen. However, I worried about how long this arrangement would work for Bob.

One Saturday evening when I arrived home, as I walked into the living room where Bob was sitting in his favorite chair, he greeted me by saying, "I don't like being home alone all day." No hello, how was your day, just a clear statement of his situation.

I walked over and put my arms around him, "Are you okay? Did anything happen today that was a problem?"

"No, I just don't like being alone all day." It was becoming clear I might need to make other plans for him or stop teaching. The latter didn't seem like much of an option in the middle of the semester. I needed time to figure out what was the best solution going forward.

When I drove in the garage the next Saturday evening, I saw a Post-it Note on the inside door to the house. It was from my neighbor Teresa. Although she knew about Bob's condition, she was not aware that I was away teaching for the day. My heart sank, thinking something horrible had happened. The note said: "Bob's at our house. He's ok."

I dropped my notebooks and papers on the kitchen counter and ran up the street to Teresa's. I only knocked once—she opened the door and quickly put her arm around me, saying, "Bob is just fine. There's nothing to worry about." She already knew I would be frightened at finding the note. I could see him sitting in their living room, hands folded in his lap, waiting patiently. He turned to look at me without a smile or recognition. I could sense that he was still anxious about whatever had transpired.

I thanked Teresa and, seeing that she was starting to prepare dinner, I said to Bob, "Come on, sweetie. Let's go home." As we walked the block to our house, I began slowly to ask Bob about his day. I was still distressed that after my long teaching day, I had come home to the remnants of a problem.

Despite my careful questioning, Bob couldn't tell me about the day in a way that made sense, but I was able to understand some of what happened. He had taken a nap in the afternoon, and when he awakened, he was confused and upset. He couldn't remember where I was and didn't know when I would return. He never looked at the note on the kitchen island, which might have reminded him of the day's plan. His anxiety increased to the point that he couldn't stay in the house. He finally decided to go to Teresa's house and see if anybody was home. He was relieved when Teresa answered the door. She calmed him with a cup of tea. He said he felt safer than when he was home alone. He told her he didn't know where I was or when I would be back.

I reassured him he had done the right thing by going to Teresa's and suggested we start dinner. I knew that getting the evening meal on the table would put us back in our evening routine, and Bob might be able to relax and put the day behind him.

While I was cleaning up the kitchen after dinner, I had time to think about the day and Bob's anxiety. I decided that I would prepare additional cards of the Saturday schedule and place them in the bathroom and bedroom, in addition to the kitchen. I hoped that he would find the plan without having to remember to return to the kitchen. I also vowed to find the time in my schedule to figure out a way for him not to be alone all day. I was so relieved our neighbors knew about Bob's memory problems and could provide him comfort and safety. If we had decided to keep it a secret, I hate to think how much worse an outcome I would have found upon my return home that day.

CHAPTER 8

The Importance of Finding Resources

At the time Bob was diagnosed with MCI, I was not aware of the importance of daily routines and activities outside the home for people with memory problems. The physicians we had seen offered no information about the importance of socializing and regular exercise. No one cautioned me about the dangers of Bob wanting to stay home alone (referred to as dementia patients wanting to isolate). Even the Alzheimer's Disease Center had brochures only for living facilities, not organizations providing programs for memory-impaired people.

As Bob reduced his volunteer activities, he didn't have much on his calendar to keep him engaged with others. I was concerned that for him, especially, too much time on his hands would create a problem of boredom and maybe even mild depression. He had suffered from depression on and off over the years but had controlled it most of his life with rigorous, regular exercise. His ability to ride his bike or jog had disappeared as his balance began to decline.

Adding to his dilemma was that when he invited me to go to San Francisco for the day to visit an art exhibition, to go for a walk, or to travel to Calistoga for lunch on the patio of a restaurant we loved, my work made me unavailable, and that distressed me too. But because I liked my work, I never thought about reducing my hours or taking early retirement. We didn't know anyone in a similar situation: wife working, husband retired. Most of our friends were still working full-time.

With some combination of love, hope, and desperation, I began regularly to scour the local newspaper for announcements of activities that might interest Bob. One evening after dinner in March of 2003, I saw a small announcement in our paper for a new class called "Mind Boosters." There was no mention of Alzheimer's in the ad. It was described as a once a week activity class for people having some memory problems. I later learned the more precise name was early stage memory loss. Only a phone number was listed for further contact. When I told Bob about it and offered to call the next day to find out the details, he quickly answered, "Sure."

I was grateful for his positive response, which I considered to be a function of his outgoing personality. I didn't want him to think I was shoving him out of the house or taking over his calendar. Neither of my concerns turned out to be valid.

I called the next day and learned that Mind Boosters had been recently developed by Adult Day Services (Adult Day). The people I spoke with were friendly and encouraging—just what I needed to encourage Bob to sign up if he was reluctant to try it.

"Everything about the class seems perfect for you. It meets on Fridays, starts on April 11, begins at 11:30, includes lunch, and you can drive to the meeting location. There's a small fee, so we'll make sure you have some cash with you." He seemed pleased to have a new place to go and that he could drive himself there.

Later, I noticed on his large desk calendar that on April 11 he had written: "Mind Boosters group in Napa without Cheri." I didn't know if he had written the note as merely a reminder for himself or a sign of concern about going alone.

After Bob came home from the first class, I couldn't wait to ask how he liked it. I knew he didn't like to be "grilled" (as he used to call it) when he first came in the door, so I held my inquiry as long as I could. Finally, I asked, "So, how was it?"

"Okay," he said, as he headed to the back of the house to change clothes. Oh no, I thought. I'm going to have to dig carefully to get real information, wait a bit more, and remember I'm not at work where my questions were viewed as a sign of healthy interest.

My work habit as a consultant was to ask lots of questions since I was usually meeting people in a business that was new to me. And I frequently needed information to work on the project after I left their office. This probing habit was hard for me to break.

I waited to ask more questions until I heard him in our bedroom. As I walked in, he offered, "There were only three other people there: two guys and a woman and another woman who taught the class." He added that he liked Kristin. She was the Program Manager and leader of the Mind Boosters program.

My brain immediately went to worrying the class wouldn't last. "Are they going to continue to have it with such a small group?"

"I guess so," he said and headed for the bathroom. This time I didn't follow him, but I wanted to hear more. I was beginning to realize, since his diagnosis, how much more time it took for him to express himself. Bob had never been a fast talker. I used to tease him that he should join the "Slow Talkers of America" club. I didn't tease him about this anymore and was trying to be more patient while he found the words he wanted.

I needn't have worried about the class closing down. Not only did the meetings continue with that small beginning group, but it also grew to about a dozen people, mostly men. He was expected there every Friday, and he quickly made new friends who, as he said, "...have the same problems as I do." I knew this meant the early difficulties of finding the right words for casual conversation.

Mind Boosters provided activities I could never have offered at home and provided memory exercises for the participants' brains, working individually, in pairs, or as one large group. One group exercise was to have the participants make as many words as they could out of a longer word. On holidays, to help keep the minds of the participants in the present and draw from old memories, the facilitator would start the exercise by writing the name of the holiday (for example "Christmas") across the top of a blank white easel pad. The participants then tried to come up with as many words with those letters as they could. The facilitator wrote the words they offered on the page, and the participants could see the list grow longer as they found more and more words. It was fun, made them work their brains, and gave them a sense of accomplishment.

The predictable routine was part of what made Mind Boosters appealing to Bob and others. The activities were varied, but the structure of the day was consistent. They knew what to expect at every session. The program started at 11:30, followed by a walk to one of several low-cost restaurants. The walk provided them with fresh air and a bit of exercise before their meal. Bob, who loved to exercise and eat, especially enjoyed this part of the program. After returning from lunch, there were exercises on paper to stimulate their memories until 2:30 when the day ended.

His first friend was a man named Gene, whom Bob frequently told me about. Gene was in his eighties and initially reached out to Bob. As their friendship grew, Gene invited Bob to join a barbershop chorus. He would drive to our house to give Bob a ride to chorus practice, as it was in the evening, and Bob didn't usually drive when it was dark. Gene always had the same comment for Bob: "You're a card, and you need to be dealt with!" Bob and I laughed about that for years.

One time when Bob was ill with the flu, Gene called to see how he was doing. I spoke with him, and at the end of the call, Gene said, "Tell Bob, I love him." Even though Bob wasn't feeling well, when I told him Gene called, he perked up and wanted to know what Gene said. I repeated Gene's closing comment: "Tell Bob, I love him."

I could see tears in Bob's eyes. He said, "I've never had a friend like Gene. All my friends in business were men always wanting to compete. Gene's just not like that."

Bob looked forward to Mind Boosters every week. Upon awakening on Friday, he'd say, "Is today Friday?" I would confirm it was, and then he'd always say, "Am I going to Mind Boosters today?"

One day, after months in the program, upon arriving home he announced, "They always go to the Chinese restaurant. I wish they would change it more often." I didn't ask if he had posed his suggestion to Kristin, something he would have done years earlier; I had already seen his assertiveness decrease since his diagnosis.

I asked, "Do you want me to call Kristin and see what the deal is about lunch?" He thought that was a good idea.

A few days later, after I talked to Kristin, I reported to Bob. "It turns out that they vote every Friday on where they want to go to lunch. Kristin said since you arrive late, they've already voted by the time you get there." I knew Bob had a hard time organizing himself to get to places on time, so I wasn't surprised by her explanation.

Bob's face showed he was indeed surprised. He reluctantly admitted that maybe getting there earlier would allow him to influence the restaurant selection. He had always struggled with punctuality, but the decline in the planning and organizing part of his brain (called executive function) was adding to this challenge. With the weekly vote about lunch, Mind Boosters allowed Bob to work on his punctuality — a side benefit to the program I never anticipated.

The first year at holiday time, Kristin invited caregivers to join the Mind Boosters participants in a party. Caregivers were asked to bring a dessert as a contribution to the festivities. I looked forward to this opportunity: a social event on a manageable scale where I might meet other caregivers. Kristin provided party hats for everyone and holiday decorations to make the plain room festive.

We four caregivers were all relatives of the participants: Gene's wife, another woman divorced from her husband along with her adult son, one husband, and me. Although I was curious to meet the other caregivers, the occasion felt a bit like a cocktail party of strangers. The only thing we had in common was the disease of our loved one. No one seemed comfortable talking about symptoms or how we were dealing with our challenges. We made small talk until the desserts were passed around. That gave us a conversation topic. "This looks wonderful. Who made this? Is it strawberry or raspberry?" At last, we were talking.

After dessert, Kristin spontaneously asked Bob and Gene if they wanted to sing a holiday song. She was aware they were attending the local barbershop chorus. I could tell by the look on Bob's face they had not practiced for this occasion, so it was great to see him willing to stand in front of the group and shyly start to sing. In his red Christmas vest, arm in arm with Gene, their rendition of Jingle Bells brought smiles to the faces of everyone.

After the singing, Kristin asked everyone, now sitting quietly, if anyone had anything they wanted to say. Then one of the caregiver wives raised her hand. With Kristin's encouragement, finally, she timidly said, "There is no shame in having Alzheimer's?" She had meant the sentence as a statement, but I heard a question in it. During the silence that followed, I felt as if she were searching for reassurance about her own feelings of shame, while the rest of us considered our feelings. Kristin rescued us all, assuring her she was right; it was a disease and no one's fault. Another quiet interval settled over the group. It was the first time I even considered that the word shame might occur in the same sentence with Alzheimer's.

In time, Bob let me know he wasn't confident enough to drive himself to Mind Boosters, so I took on the transportation duties. Friday still provided a welcome break for me. I could catch my breath, take a nap, and generally restore my energies to continue to meet the demands of his illness and the needs of my clients.

Through Mind Boosters, Bob found friendship, mental challenges, and fun. I had a four-hour break from caregiving and Bob had a place to go every Friday. It was an essential resource for both of us.

CHAPTER 9

Challenges in Support Group

A short time after our interviews for the dual support group, Evelyn, the social worker, telephoned to invite us to join the weekly Monday morning support groups in Santa Rosa, one for Bob and one for me. I readily accepted, thanked her, and asked for directions. I calculated the trip would take an hour each way in good traffic.

Bob seemed pleased when I told him the news. After years of going to his office to start the business week, he liked having somewhere, anywhere, to go on Monday mornings. Our commitment was for eight weeks.

I made a plan to get him up earlier than usual for our first meeting. It was beginning to take him longer to dress, and I was still getting used to planning the extra time he needed to accomplish personal care tasks. Furthermore, I'd driven this two-lane route many times and knew that unpredictable traffic could add time to our trip.

The weekend before the initial meetings, a knot formed in my stomach every time I thought of the drive and the unknowns. I worried about all kinds of possibilities: What if Bob didn't like the group and walked out? What if people in my group were critical of my caregiving? What if, what if, what if? Bob, however, showed no signs of similar concerns.

Traffic on the two-lane roads was light (one anxiety diminished), and we arrived at our destination with minutes to spare. As we walked through the parking lot, I sensed some apprehension in Bob, who acted a bit confused. I reached for his hand, knowing that touch always settled him. When we entered the building, I saw to my left the room with an open door where his group was meeting and pointed it out. "There's your meeting, sweetie. Mine must be around the corner, so I'll see you in about an hour and a half."

"Aren't you coming with me?" he asked.

I had not counted on this reaction from him. I repeated what the arrangement was. "There are two meetings. One for caregivers, which is the one I'm going to. Then there is this one for people who are having memory problems. This is your meeting." I pointed to the open door as I crossed my fingers that his reluctance would fade with my explanation.

Slowly, he turned toward the open door and walked inside. His hesitance reminded me of a small boy on the first day of school when he didn't know anyone and everything was new. But as soon as the therapist saw him and greeted him by name, he stepped toward her and shook her hand, never turning around to say goodbye to me. I felt he was in good hands.

Down the hallway, I saw a restroom and darted in thinking I would be better off to be a bit late for my first meeting with strangers than excuse myself mid-meeting to find a toilet. But to my surprise, as soon as the door closed behind me, I burst into tears. Worrying about Bob was becoming a habit, but I had not realized I was also anxious about this first for me: talking to strangers about complicated feelings I was having about the changes in Bob.

My cry was over quickly, fortunately without witnesses. I wiped my face and looked in the mirror. Did I look as frazzled as I felt? I decided not to worry about my appearance, the opposite of the care I took when going to a new client's office for the first time.

When I walked into the meeting room, Sharon, the other social worker from our interview day, was talking to one of the six other participants, who sat in an informal circle. She turned toward me with a warm smile and extended her hand in welcome. I was relieved, not only to be where I felt I was supposed to be but reassured by Sharon's friendly manner. She quickly introduced me to each caregiver in the group. "You came to the right place," one of the women responded. "We're glad you're here."

Then Sharon started the meeting with an announcement. One of the caregivers who had been part of the group, but absent today, would no longer be attending. Instead, she was finding a facility for her husband. He had later stage Alzheimer's symptoms, including aggressive sexual advances that had become dangerous to her as well as unbearable. Out of respect for the caregiver, Sharon did not go into any detail about the husband's behavior. I had read about aggressive behavior in Alzheimer's patients and knew that it was not something that usually happened in the early stages of a dementia disease. I never imagined that Bob would be dangerous to me. He was such a gentle guy and had never been hostile or inappropriate with me or others.

The people in the group seemed more saddened than shocked by the news and offered their sympathy. In a reassuring manner, Sharon answered a few questions about the caregiver, then moved the group to focus on our situations by asking, "Who would like to check in first? Let's see what's been going on in your world."

Everyone settled into their chairs and seemed ready. Sharon turned to me and said, "Since you're new to the group, Cheri, would you like to listen to the others today? You may not want to say anything, and that's just fine. Please do what's comfortable for you."

It was so thoughtful of her. I immediately felt relieved to be able to take in others' stories and not be concerned about what I would or wouldn't say. She turned to the man sitting next to her and indicated he should start the "check-ins."

I was familiar with this process as I had taken courses in facilitating groups in a workplace setting. Each participant tells what significant or troubling experiences they have had since the last meeting. Sometimes they also state they would like to have more time after the check-ins to deal with a troubling issue. Because I was new, Sharon asked the others, mostly caregivers for their spouses, to begin with a brief history of their caregiving experience. She also explained to me that their loved ones all had been diagnosed with Alzheimer's disease, except for one whose spouse had frontotemporal dementia (a condition I knew nothing about).

Sharon managed the discussion to provide time for everyone. When she turned to me— the last person in the circle—she asked if I wanted to say anything. Because I felt on the edge of being able to keep my emotions under control, I said very little. I explained about Bob's recent diagnosis and what memory difficulties I had already noticed in him. A couple of people commented on how unusually cooperative it was that Bob was open to finding out about his memory problems so early. Although I had heard this re-mark before, it reminded me how proud I was of him. I couldn't say anything in response, and then we were out of time. I knew this first meeting would be the hardest and told myself the next time would be more comfortable.

I headed down the hall to find Bob before he could go outside and perhaps not remember where we had parked. As it happened, his entire group had emptied into the hall-way. At first, I could not spot him but then saw him talking with another fellow. When Bob saw me, he smiled broadly. He looked calm and cheerful. I gave him a wave and felt myself begin to relax.

I asked how he liked his group as we drove home. He responded with how much he liked the therapist and how helpful she was in introducing him to the group and mak-ing him feel welcome.

Then he added, "They don't talk very much." I asked him to say more about their discussion. He explained they only talked when the therapist asked them a question. And many times, their answers were a simple "Yes" or "No." I reassured him that as they got to know him, they might speak more. He didn't disagree.

That was the sum of our conversation. We were both fa-tigued from our first group meeting. Bob's new habit of turning to silence was something I was trying to get used to. As the weeks went by, Bob's concerns increased about the lack of contribution from other people in the group. He was having difficulty connecting with them. My theory was incorrect that once they knew each other, the conversation would improve. Bob thought that the facilitator should have ways to make people talk more.

Only later did I learn, when Bob began to have difficulty with his own speech, why the others in the group might have been so uncommunicative. It wasn't that they didn't want to say something; they probably were unable to find the words to say anything.

Meanwhile, in my caregivers' group, I began to open up more and spoke about my frustrations. At this stage, Bob was losing things, forgetting appointments, promising to take care of errands and then not doing them. It felt like more and more was being dumped on me, not by agreement, but by what I sometimes saw as irresponsible behavior.

One day I told the group about a recent incident with Bob. I had asked Bob to pick up the cleaning. He said he would. Back home at the end of the day, when I checked to see where the cleaning was, he admitted he hadn't picked it up. This kind of mistake was getting to be the norm, I added. Bob would sign up for a task to help me out, then forget or claim he was confused about it. Rarely did he have an apology.

I announced, "I'm so tired of his making commitments he doesn't keep." My frustration in reciting such memories made me start to cry. One of the husband caregivers said, "Well, Cheri, in the past he wouldn't do it, but now he can't. That's a big difference you have to accept."

In the silence that followed, I did not respond, but my mind was on fire. With the word "wouldn't," the man had hit a nerve larger than he could have realized. In the years before Bob was diagnosed, he sometimes did not follow through on responsibilities. This behavior had led to many difficult conversations as we tried to sort out where the problem lay. It finally came to light that when the task involved some reminder of either his first marriage or his upbringing, he reacted with a kind of stubbornness that left me upset. The man's use of the word "can't" hit another nerve; do I have to accept that Bob's lack of follow-through will continue?

Finally, it was someone else's turn to talk, but I wasn't able to listen. I sat there feeling sorry for myself and waiting for the meeting to be over.

I thought about that man's comment a hundred times. The first twenty times, I had a good argument: he was out of line in making such judgments about circumstances he knew little about. His advice came across as instruction to me, with no empathy. Slowly, though, I began to come to terms with the truth in the word "can't." Bob couldn't do many things anymore. Believing that he was irresponsible or stubborn just kept me angry. If not for the group, how much longer would it have taken me to find and accept the hard truth about Bob's situation and still love and care for him? This particularly big adjustment, though, like others, meant that I had to find a way to accept the reality of more responsibilities.

Bob and I completed two eight-week sessions in the Santa Rosa group, but then we decided to search for a dual support group closer to home. For me, despite the benefits of a certain unwelcome piece of advice, many caregivers had been dealing with the challenges of the disease for some time and were experiencing more complicated issues than Bob and I were. (My thoughts went back to Evelyn's comments all those weeks ago about putting us in a cancer ward when we had just been given a diagnosis.) And Bob had begun to complain regularly about not being able to connect with the people in his group.

An additional difficulty was that when there was a holiday, the two groups of patients and caregivers sometimes planned a social activity in place of a meeting. They organized barbecues on Saturday afternoons, for example. Not only was it just too far for us to drive for a social outing, I frequently had other business responsibilities. Bob and I knew we were missing essential benefits, such as making friends with people who understood our situation, but the lack of a good fit for Bob and social outings we could not attend anyway, plus the travel distance, eased us into the decision to leave the groups.

I gave notice to Sharon that we would not be continuing with the next session. She was understanding and gracefully offered me her appreciation for our participation. I then began our search for another dual support group by contacting Adult Day. Bob and I needed groups, not only closer to home but more appropriate to our separate needs. I was beginning to learn that finding resources to meet our requirements took time and energy; the first attempt didn't always work.

This first support group experience certainly helped me see a hard truth: What other caregivers suggest may be challenging to hear, yet helpful in the long run. I was beginning to learn that patience was a requirement for many parts of my new life.

CHAPTER 10

Finding Humor in Repetition

I had heard that a typical dementia behavior was the repetition of simple questions about daily living. And I had heard an elderly caregiver at Adult Day ask, "Why does my husband ask the same question over and over?" As she described her struggle to cope with her husband's new habit, I thought that repetition would not be that difficult for me. I would call on the patience I used as a teacher when distracted students asked a question I had just answered. I'm not sure I was a patient teacher, but that was the picture I had of myself. And of course, I hadn't experienced that kind of repetition from Bob—yet.

My support group did teach me to expect questions such as, "Have we had lunch?" And I was told Bob might ask the whereabouts of a relative who had died. So I was on the lookout for such questions, but I also had dozens of happy memories of Bob's ability to use repetition as a way to create humor. He had an uncanny way of introducing repetitive behavior when no one was expecting it and usually got a laugh. Even though I had never been around someone funny in this way, I enjoyed his unique humor.

Before Bob became ill, my parents, who lived in Washington State, visited us about once a year. They came by train, and we would pick them up at the Amtrak train station in Martinez, the county seat of a county south of us. It was no Grand Central; arrival and departure times were imprecise.

On the day my parents were to leave, Bob and I took them back to the station early, allowing time for variations in the departure schedule. Standing on the platform of the small old-fashioned station, trying to find something to do to pass the time, after a five-day visit, was sometimes difficult. Not for Bob. He found a rusty rail spike somewhere along the tracks. We all admired it as if it were an antique. Then he accidentally dropped it on the cement platform in front of the station. It made such a loud clang; we all jumped in surprise and then laughed. A few minutes later he dropped it again, this time on purpose. My mother and I laughed, knowing Bob was playing a grade school trick and trying to entertain us. The look on his face told me I was right. My father, however, lost interest; his sense of humor didn't include silliness. But Bob continued to drop the spike every few minutes until I begged him to stop. He loved making us laugh but knew when the joke had run its course.

I had experienced this side of Bob's sense of humor for years. When we lived in the Bay Area, there was an outdated diner on College Avenue in Berkeley which he told me was a greasy spoon and never to eat there. For years, when we were driving nearby, he would start to warn me we were coming near a critical site. I would always say, "I know it's that greasy spoon."

"No, this is a place you don't know," he would retort. He would persist and act as if it were something else. When we finally drove by the diner, he would announce, "There it is—that diner is a real greasy spoon!" I would burst into laughter and so would he. It was silly, but we loved the game.

Such games were well-integrated into our daily lives until Bob became ill. Then the trivial repetition only appeared when I started it. On a good day, he could go along and enjoy the old back and forth. Some days, though, the result was more confusion than fun.

On Super Bowl Sunday, about two years into Bob's disease, while cleaning up after breakfast, I asked him, "Do you want to come to the NFL Super Bowl party today?" There was no party planned, but we had both had miserable histories attending them and liked to joke about such parties. This time, he looked at me quizzically. I assured him there wasn't a party, and his face relaxed with a smile. But later in the day, when I turned on the television, I again asked if he wanted to come to watch the New England Patriots and Carolina Panthers at the Super Bowl party. He laughed out loud and plopped down next to me on the living room couch. It was wonderful to see the playful Bob I had known for so long enjoy our old joke routine again.

After the game, he said he was going to lie down for a nap. In those days, he had begun to take a nap almost every afternoon. As he was leaving the living room, he turned and asked, "Is it okay to lie down on top of the electric blanket?" He hadn't started asking me the "Have we had lunch?" questions, but he had asked me this question many, many times. And he didn't mean the repetition as a joke. I decided to give up explaining that it wasn't good for the blanket. I didn't want to lose the fun we'd been having by showing him my irritation at this same question. Sometimes I made the mistake of turning my negative feelings inward, only later remembering his disease was the culprit.

I stood up, put my arms around him, and asked, "Do you have any idea how many times you've asked me that?" He shook his head no. I said, "Two to three times a week times 52 weeks times two years—about 300 times." After the words were out of my mouth, I realized my sentence had a touch of sarcasm that might hurt his feelings. But he started to laugh and so did I. The laughter reduced my annoyance.

We hugged each other, and he carefully walked down the hallway into what we still called the guest bedroom, though it was his bedroom now. After decades together in one bed, we had begun sleeping apart. His nocturnal bathroom trips had become so frequent that my sleep was interrupted three or four times a night. Besides, since becoming his caregiver, I just needed time alone and told him so. After he reluctantly moved to the guest bedroom, I began to sleep better.

This day, he lay down on top of the electric blanket as if we'd never talked about it. I sighed, put a small afghan over him, turned on the CD player with his favorite Mozart CD, and saw that he was almost asleep.

We probably had that electric blanket conversation another 300 times. We were lucky, though, that we could continue finding humor, including our particular brand. Along the way, I learned that finding it sometimes meant taking a risk, but there was often a reward that brought some fun to our lives and reminded me how much I loved him.

CHAPTER 11

A Bit of Hope—NPH Surgery

In the spring of 2005, Bob began to have more balance problems and difficulty walking. He was beginning to use a cane and struggled to remember where he left it after each use. While I worried less about his falling and breaking a bone or hurting himself in some other way, reminding him to take the cane with him was another notch on my ever-expanding "To Do" list. His memory was now failing him in the simplest of tasks.

His performance at follow-up visits to the Alzheimer's Disease Center and Kaiser over the prior three years was progressively worse on all of the many tests they administered. Doctors didn't offer a new diagnosis. I knew that only an autopsy could medically confirm the presence of Alzheimer's. Bob's willingness to discuss his decline, often announcing he needed assistance with something, helped me recognize the culprit must be Alzheimer's.

At the time of his increasing imbalance, we often saw television ads that promised an almost miracle cure for Alzheimer's patients who might be suffering from Normal Pressure Hydrocephalus (NPH). Since the commercial said so little about what NPH was (we later learned it's an accumulation of water in the brain), or what the procedure was, we decided to ask his primary care doctor for a referral to a neurologist to explore the possibilities. At the appointment, I was specific in my request not to see the previous neurologist. She reassured me, "Oh, he's retired. Don't worry about that."

After obtaining the referral, we were able to see a young, highly recommended neurologist. Without saying so to one another, Bob and I were both hoping for some good news for a change. The new neurologist turned out to be caring and meticulous. At the first appointment, she observed Bob's walking up and down the hall and then performed a complete neurological exam, including the Mini-Mental Status test he had taken several times by now. Afterward, she explained he might indeed be suffering from NPH, an accumulation of liquid in his brain. Memories of the black areas on his CT scan years earlier came to my mind.

She described both NPH and the procedure in understandable terms: A shunt (a hollow tube) would be implanted in his brain. The tube would carry the excess spinal fluid down into his abdominal cavity. Nothing would show on the surface of his body. With less pressure from the excess water, his walking and cognition might be improved. Since she was not a neurosurgeon, we would need a referral to one.

She went on to explain that if Bob wanted to proceed with the possibility of surgery, she needed to prove that specific symptoms were present: problems with balance, urinary incontinence, and dementia. In my opinion, Bob was struggling with all three. However, any neurosurgeon would first require that these symptoms be confirmed. She added a warning: There was a risk during the surgery that a patient might have a stroke. The word "stroke" was a shock to me. I looked at Bob to see if he was distressed by this warning. He seemed unfazed, so I asked the neurologist what the next step would be.

The answer was a spinal tap. The procedure would prove if withdrawing some fluid from Bob's spine in the lumbar region would reduce the pressure on his brain just enough to improve his balance. As we learned, the spinal tap was a preliminary test. If Bob walked better after the procedure, then the NPH surgery might create the same improvement. Less fluid on his brain would equal less pressure, which would equal better balance and an even more important outcome: better cognition.

She also warned us that after the spinal tap, Bob might experience a headache for several days, as well as nausea, dizziness, and back pain. She added that I would be welcome to stay in the room to observe while she performed the procedure. I was relieved I would be able to stay with him during the spinal tap. We made an appointment to return the next week for the procedure.

The whole process of inserting the needle in his back and withdrawing the fluid was over in about 15 minutes. Bob was a cooperative patient and must have felt confident in her as he was quiet and calm. After she finished, she asked him to get down from the table carefully and walk up and down the hallway while she observed him. My fingers crossed, I stood behind her and watched as well. His walk looked steadier to me, but I also knew that I wanted it to be better and that Bob usually performed well on any test.

When we all returned to the exam room, the doctor pronounced him a possible candidate for the surgery. It seemed like good news. It was the first opportunity, perhaps, to improve some of Bob's problems. She would send her findings (in essence, a recommendation) to the neurosurgeon, but we would be at the mercy of the surgeon's decision as to whether he would be willing to perform the surgery.

Our first referral was to a neurosurgeon at a Kaiser medical center in Sacramento, an hour to the north of Napa. We were both optimistic about the referral. When the appointment day arrived, I drove us while trying to keep my expectations under control.

We arrived on time, but my hopes were diminished when the neurosurgeon, a middle-aged man, came into the waiting room. He was unfriendly, and he brusquely told me I would have to stay in the waiting room. "I need to see the patient alone," was his only explanation.

Having accompanied Bob to appointments for years, I found this attitude offensive. Furthermore, Kaiser's philosophy was to include family members in most appointments. This restriction was a first, and I was disappointed. The surgeon must have thought I would somehow try to speak for Bob to influence his assessment.

In less than ten minutes, the neurosurgeon retrieved me from the waiting room. As soon as he closed the exam room door, he turned to me and abruptly announced that he was not willing to do the surgery. He said Bob would not benefit from it. When I asked why, he responded, "As soon as we came into the exam room, Mr. Jacobs made a joke. Anyone who can do that does not meet the cognitive decline requirement."

I was astonished and angry. I knew that despite Bob's ability to make a joke, the tasks he couldn't do were too numerous to count. I tried in vain to tell the doctor how Bob struggled with walking and increasingly poor memory. My argument went nowhere. The surgeon defended his decision by declaring that too many neurologists thought a shunt was the answer to Alzheimer's. He held to his decision and said he would not perform the surgery. He opened the door and indicated that it was the end of the visit. Bob and I left feeling disappointed and dejected.

The next day I called our empathetic neurologist to tell her what had transpired. She said, "Don't worry. I will refer you to another neurosurgeon in Redwood City. I think he will be more open to the surgery." While Bob and I waited for the next appointment to be arranged, we continued to talk about how important it was for us to pursue something that might help. I was concerned about the amount of time the appointments were taking from my work, but I was trying hard not to show that frustration to Bob. He deserved all the support I could muster.

A couple of weeks later, the appointment set, I drove 75 miles south to the Kaiser medical center in Redwood City to see another neurosurgeon. The facility was large and finding the neurosurgery department complicated. Bob followed me somewhat bewildered but still positive about the appointment.

In contrast to the Sacramento neurosurgeon, this one, also a man, treated us both with care and respect. I immediately felt comfortable and optimistic. After examining Bob and looking at his CT scans, he announced that he thought Bob was a good candidate for the surgery.

Along with that good news, he repeated the risks, including that a stroke in the middle of the surgery was a possibility. Again, the prospect of a stroke filled me with worry, but I couldn't tell if Bob comprehended what a stroke might mean with his current health challenges. The surgeon also showed us a video demonstrating the surgery and suggested we go home and take the time we needed in order to make the surgery decision.

Once again at home, Bob struggled with understanding what the surgery would be like. He asked me over and over, "Should I do it?" Despite his impairments, I wanted it to be his decision. When I reminded him that the surgeon in Redwood City had said, "We can't promise anything, Bob, but if you were my pop, I'd say go ahead and have the surgery. We don't have anything else to offer you." The word "pop" did it for him. Bob's children had always called him "Pop" and that familiar term gave him confidence that the surgeon had his best interests at heart. He finally decided to have the surgery and for a uniquely personal reason.

With the surgery scheduled for early morning, we drove to Redwood City the night before and stayed at a nearby motel where fortunately, Kaiser had made arrangements for family members to receive a discounted rate. I would be spending a second night there too, while Bob stayed in the hospital.

Bob was nervous the evening before the surgery and asked me if I thought he was doing the right thing. I reassured him that he had made the best decision, given there were no other choices to improve his situation. Because he seemed anxious, we decided to go to bed early and get a good night's sleep.

Upon arrival at the hospital the next morning, Bob was quickly taken into the prep area. I was told I'd be called to join him when he was ready for the surgery. However, it turned out the medical team was running late that day, so he didn't go into surgery until almost three hours after the scheduled time. Unaware of the delay, I sat by myself in a waiting room for family members for what seemed like forever. The longer I waited, the more anxious I became. I began to imagine that Bob had a stroke during the procedure.

Our surgeon poked his head in the waiting room in the late afternoon and gave me a thumbs-up sign. He apologized for the delay, acknowledged it must have caused me extra worry, and then assured me the surgery had gone well. There had been no stroke, and Bob was in the recovery room. I would be able to see him in a couple of hours. He explained that until Bob was up and around, we wouldn't know how much the shunt would help.

Nonetheless, because of the surgeon's comforting manner, I felt some temporary optimism. I went outside, bought myself a take-out dinner, ate it at the motel, and lay down to relax before returning to the hospital. My optimism was tenuous, though. The hours alone allowed me to worry about everything. Much later, I realized I would have benefited from asking someone to come with me.

At about 8:00 that evening, almost twelve hours after I had delivered him to the surgery prep area, I was finally able to go to Bob's hospital room. He looked exhausted and fragile in the hospital bed; it was hard for me to be upbeat. No one's appearance is improved by a hospital gown, but he looked especially small and child-like in the hospital bed with tubes coming out of his arms. His hair was greasy and uncombed, and he needed a shave. The handsome man I had known for so many years was missing.

He was awake but seemed to be in a bad mood, which was unusual for him. When I bent down to kiss him on the cheek, he barely responded. Then he said he had a terrible headache and was worried about finding his glasses.

In addition, the noise in the ward was deafening. The conversations of other families were loud, plus a television's volume was turned on high. I just wanted to put Bob in a wheelchair and take him home. Of course, that wasn't an option. Instead, I asked a nurse to get Bob some medicine for his headache and to lower the volume on the TV blaring from the other patient's bed. When I asked about his glasses, she said she had no idea where they might be and walked away. I tried not to worry about the glasses but was concerned that he would have a sleepless night. I left as soon as he took the Tylenol. It had been a long day for both of us.

The next day his headache had not diminished. The staff was concerned about releasing him prematurely. In the end, they kept him another three days, two days longer than expected. Still, I was told not to worry. Having struggled with migraines since I was a child, I knew what serious headache pain was. I could wait.

Finally, on the afternoon of day four, Bob was discharged. He was relieved to go home and struggled with the headache off and on for the next couple of weeks. I alerted his surgeon and learned that the headache might take a while to disappear, but there was nothing to be concerned about.

As long as Bob was living with the headache pain and spending time in bed, his reluctance to walk meant I could not determine if the surgery had helped his balance. I tried to nurse him with good food and reassurance that things would get better.

Eventually, the headaches waned, and he resumed attending Mind Boosters. Our lives returned to our regular daily routine. Bob did seem to walk better, but I couldn't note any improvement in his mental capacities. I asked him from time to time if he felt his brain was working better. He couldn't answer with any certainty. He was only able to tell me he felt depressed.

One day he confessed to me he couldn't stop thinking about dying. All I could do was hold him and reassure him I was there for him. I called the neurosurgeon and relayed Bob's concerns. He suggested an appointment to adjust the amount of liquid the shunt drained from the brain. We returned to the Redwood City hospital several times in the next few months for such adjustments. Finally, the neurosurgeon explained that additional modifications would probably do no good. The shunt was less effective than we had allowed ourselves to hope.

Although we both had known that significant improvement was a long shot, now we had to accept that his memory was no better and the same cognitive issues remained. And in a few months, his balance problems returned.

Meanwhile, within a month of the surgery, I faced the fact that I felt burned out. The idea of a vacation began to occur to me. How about Hawaii? Even thinking about the touch of trade winds on my skin and the spotted doves cooing in the palm fronds soothed me. I began dreaming that I would be able to relax and recoup some energy and decided to talk with Bob about our getting away. Of course, arranging a trip would take time and effort. I would not stop taking care of Bob the whole time, but I knew I had to do something for me too. As it happened, there was no reason to spell out my needs to Bob. I didn't have to; he liked the idea when I said I would reserve the same condo we had stayed in once before on the Big Island.

Finally, we both had something to look forward to.

CHAPTER 12

Getting Help at Home

Taking a trip to the Big Island of Hawaii seemed like a just reward following Bob's surgery. The Big Island was a paradise with fewer tourists and small towns that made the island look like it was the 1950s. Our condo was large and inviting. Everything was perfect, except Bob. His balance problems returned to the point that I rented a wheelchair for him and tried without success to help him relax and enjoy our day trips around the island. I came home more tired than I left. Something had to change.

Letting anyone besides my closest friends know I was beginning to struggle with my increasing responsibilities was very different—and difficult. In my work life, it had always been easy to assign others to assist with a project or think through a business problem with me. However, Bob's illness was somehow a different situation for me. When friends and acquaintances asked how Bob was doing, I usually gave them a short answer and then changed the subject.

It felt like an admission of failure if I answered honestly to a common question from clients, "How are you doing?"

In addition, my feelings about help were ever-changing: I want help; I don't need it; I don't want to ask for it; I especially don't want to supervise someone who is helping. Doesn't getting help mean I'm not a capable spouse and caregiver?

Finally, I decided I needed to seek professional help to come to grips with my reluctance to get assistance with my growing responsibilities. It was reassuring to remember that therapy had been a benefit to me at various times in my life. I decided to make an appointment with Lynne, the therapist who had helped me years earlier deal with the shock of Bob's MCI diagnosis. I thought I would feel safe in telling Lynne how troubled I was. I was confident she wouldn't launch into the most common suggestion I was accustomed to hearing: "If you need help, just hire someone."

I started to feel better just having made an appointment with her. When I entered her serene and comfortable office, I plopped down on the tan leather couch and declared, more or less in these words, "I have to do everything. Bob used to pay all the bills and manage our investments. Now it's up to me. All grocery shopping is my responsibility. I'm doing the majority of meal preparation and cleanup. I have to arrange his medical and dental appointments and then take him to them as well. The whole thing is a logistical nightmare because I'm also trying to be available for my clients and keep those relationships humming along. It's too much, and I don't think he even notices I'm now responsible for everything."

By the time I got the last sentence out, tears were running down my cheeks. I then sat in a despondent pout for a few minutes while Lynne patiently waited for me to gather myself. She finally asked, "What do you think you'd like to do about it?"

Her question annoyed me. Here was another task for me to accomplish: Figure out what to do about having to do everything. It might have been funny in a class on Time Management or Getting Yourself Organized but not there that day. By the end of the session, feeling better after venting my frustrations, I told Lynne I would think about what I might like to do.

I continued to balk at friends' specific suggestions to get help with household chores or find someone to be with Bob for a few hours, or both. I even developed logical reasons that hiring any help was not an answer. The main reason, I told myself, was that when I started my consulting business, I vowed I would never hire employees. In corporate life, I had done my share of hiring, firing, and supervising. Since I was going to advise other business owners about their employee problems, I surely didn't want to have employees of my own to contend with. And I had to admit to myself that I didn't like the idea of a stranger in our house alone with Bob.

I continued to talk about my situation with Lynne, and then she gave me an idea I felt I could try. Its advantage was that it did not involve anyone working at the house. She told me that when she was writing her Ph.D. thesis, she asked her babysitter to make a large casserole or a pot of hearty soup once a week. Soon, she received two or three nights of nutritious meals without having to interrupt her writing to prepare it. She suggested I casually put out the word that I was looking for someone to provide a similar dinner once a week. I put her suggestion to work right away and began to tell everyone I met with or ran into that

I was looking for someone to prepare food once a week for Bob and me. It worked too.

Within a month, my neighbor Betty told me about a woman she knew who might be starting a home-cooked meal delivery service. Soon I arranged to meet Chris at our house. When she arrived, I introduced her to Bob, and the three of us chatted informally. From the moment she arrived, she was friendly, easily volunteering information about her love of cooking. She told us she prepared meals for her family gatherings and knew how to cook a wide variety of foods. She seemed to understand our situation and agreed to try out the weekly meal service. It was a perfect fit.

Chris began bringing a full dinner on Tuesday nights. The portions were so generous, I was usually able to stretch them into three dinners. The weekly deliveries included homemade soup, a hot vegetable dish, an entrée, and a dessert. On holidays, Chris made a traditional meal related to the holiday and included a special dessert along with fancy holiday napkins, just for fun. Bob loved her cooking and so did I. More valuable to me was knowing that a great tasting dinner would appear like clockwork in the middle of the week.

I shared my good news with Lynne, who encouraged me to use this experience to build my confidence and get additional help. About the same time, I had begun to understand that Bob's whole body would be affected by the changes in his brain. I was already seeing his difficulties with balance and walking, especially up and down stairs. The obvious answer, one I was getting closer to accepting, was to hire a caregiver to help Bob and simultaneously give me a break.

Shortly after that, during a meeting for caregivers at Adult Day, I listened to a woman relate a story about being unable to go to an evening concert with a friend. Her husband was in the late stages of Alzheimer's, and she said she couldn't leave him alone. When someone suggested she have a person come in to relieve her for the evening, she said, "Oh no, my husband won't let me bring anyone into the house." She admitted she was depressed about her situation but felt stuck with it.

I didn't want to end up like that. I always told Bob when I was leaving and where I was going, but I didn't have to get permission from him to leave home. Listening to that story encouraged me to think about finding a caregiver for at least part of a day, once a week. It would give me the freedom to leave him and he would be safe.

The next week I contacted a caregiver agency to hire a person to be with Bob for one morning a week. I considered it an experiment and only told Bob I had ordered a caregiver to come to the house. He had no questions when I alerted him to the plan.

It took a while to make the arrangements, as the agency did an in-home interview, and I had to complete a long questionnaire about our caregiving needs. I was encouraged by their thorough sign-up process, even though the hourly fee was expensive. The experiment was short-lived. The first caregiver seemed unable to arrive on time which made me late getting to my meetings. I asked the agency for another, more responsible caregiver. The next one was new to the job and got lost taking Bob for a drive around Napa. She resorted to asking him if he knew how to get home when she realized how lost she was. I alerted the agency I wouldn't need their services.

A month later my luck seemed to change. A friend whose husband had Alzheimer's told me about the caregiver she was using and highly recommended him. I asked for his contact information and made plans to talk to Bob about him.

I hadn't conferred with Bob about using the caregiver agency, and afterward, it felt like that was a mistake. It was a shortcut meant to save me time. I didn't want to make that mistake again. We had always talked through all our serious decisions. I especially wanted him to be in on this decision. Also, I worried that if I waited until he started to decline more, I might not be able to include him in the decision.

By now, I had learned it was best to talk to Bob in the morning. As the day went on, his energy and ability to comprehend waned. After breakfast one day, I asked if we could talk for a minute. He agreed and I began to explain, "I think it might be a good idea to have someone come in a couple of hours every week to be with you." I did not refer to the failed experience with the agency. I added it would give me a free afternoon to meet with clients, go to doctor's appointments, and run errands. I said, "I already have the name of a caregiver who comes highly recommended."

"I want it to be a guy," he quickly responded.

"This person is a guy and his name is Rudy," I happily reported. "I'd like to see if he would be available for one afternoon a week." I further explained that I knew he didn't need anyone now, but it would be good for both of us to get to know someone and establish a routine.

I watched his face to see if a frown appeared. Had I surprised him or was he expecting something like this? I couldn't read his expression. It took him a while to say anything. Finally, he responded, "Okay, let's try it."

Pleased as I was that he accepted the idea, I realized I was hoping he would give me some kudos for planning ahead, for finding someone already tested, and that this caregiver was a male. None of that seemed to impress him; he took in all the information with no visible reaction. I had to be content with the fact that he hadn't resisted and that I had taken another step to get assistance. The first step towards getting reliable outside help to stay with Bob was a big one for both of us.

Connecting with Rudy was easier than I imagined. The next day, I called him and left a message. When he called back, I introduced myself, told him how I had learned about him, and we chatted easily. I invited him to come to our house to get acquainted and see if we could work out a caregiving arrangement.

Much to my relief, Rudy arrived on time. When I opened the front door to greet him, I was impressed by his big friendly smile. He was middle-aged and shorter than Bob but looked healthy and strong. I later learned he had grown up in Mexico City. In his youth, he had been a body-builder and had won the Mr. Mexico City competition.

I showed Rudy into the living room where Bob was already seated. Bob's manners were intact; he rose to shake hands with Rudy. As we three sat down to chat, Bob was quiet, but I could tell he was using his old business interview skills, watching body language and listening carefully to what Rudy said. Rudy emphasized he was only available on Monday afternoons. It was not the best choice for us. Bob went to Mind Boosters on Friday, so I would have preferred a break mid-week, but I knew we needed to give it a try.

When I turned to Bob for his reaction, he was nodding that Monday was okay. When we walked to the front door,

I checked with Rudy about his fees and agreed on a time for him to arrive the next Monday. After he left, I walked back to Bob, still standing in the living room. I gave him a big hug and said, "I think this is going to be really good, don't you?"

He nodded, but I could feel his hesitance. We both knew that Rudy's help represented the beginning of a different stage in living with Alzheimer's (which we both now used to refer to his illness). I think Bob may have viewed the idea of Rudy as a sign of further decline in his abilities. My emotions centered on the relief that I was going to get a break one more afternoon a week.

When Monday morning came, I reminded Bob that Rudy would be there in the afternoon and that I'd be going out. He asked, "What am I supposed to do with him?" I certainly didn't expect that question. Bob didn't need help with dressing or eating, as he was still able to care for himself and always insisted that he wear casual business attire. No sweats for him. Still, his question was unexpected.

Reluctantly, I went into problem-solving mode, thinking if I could write out a list (mainly for Rudy), Bob would feel less anxious about this first afternoon. The list I wrote included various activities they could do together, including going for a walk, watching Bob's favorite video of Broadway musicals, and putting the garbage and recycling together for the next day's pick-up. I hoped the list would reassure him that I was not suggesting he was incapable of anything. I showed Bob the list and put it on the kitchen island if he needed to remind himself.

Again, Rudy arrived right on time. Despite my relief, I was nervous. The bad experience with the first caregiver didn't help. Leaving Bob in the care of someone else created more anxiety than I had anticipated. I talked nervously, probably telling Rudy more than he needed to know. I also gave him a tour of the house, explaining some of Bob's routine. At this stage, Bob was still verbal and not hesitant to say if he didn't like something. However, he was forgetful about taking his cane on a walk, so I alerted Rudy to the need for a reminder. And I reassured myself that Rudy had been a caregiver a long time for people with dementia. Bob would be in good hands.

I didn't have a client meeting that day but having some fun never entered my mind. Instead, I ran errands and felt as if I had a better handle on the week to come. When I returned late that afternoon, things seemed to have gone well. Rudy waited to leave until I came home, which was a good sign. I hadn't thought to make sure he understood he should stay until I returned.

Bob didn't jump up from the couch to tell me how great the day had been, but I saw that Rudy had brought his guitar and learned that he had played and sung "Besame Mucho." It was such a surprise to me. I knew Bob loved music of all kinds, and in our first conversation we learned that Rudy was a musician, but I had not thought of asking him to play for Bob—individual musical performances were not in my budget. I then looked at the list I had drawn up. They had accomplished everything on it—such an excellent start to this new routine.

In the next weeks, our lives seemed to fall into a comfortable pattern. One Monday, after Rudy left, Bob told me that Rudy had talked about a musical group he performed with. When Bob asked him, "Do you have a gig this weekend?" Rudy admitted that he didn't know what "gig" meant. Bob gave him a quick lesson in how to use the word, adding that musicians considered it hip to call a performance a gig. Bob proudly announced to me that Rudy loved it and used it in every sentence he could. This sharing seemed to strengthen their growing bond.

Then things began to change. I came home early one day and found Rudy in the street by himself lining up the containers for the garbage service. He was holding the list I had written.

"Why isn't Bob helping you?" I asked as I rolled down my window and pulled the car to a stop.

He smiled and said, "It's okay. I don't mind doing it."

I pursued, "I want him to continue to do the garbage with you so he won't forget how. If you do it alone, he won't have a chance to practice." Rudy smiled again and assured me this was the best way. As I drove the car into the garage, I realized that Rudy had figured out something I had not; Bob was already beyond being able to do the garbage preparation.

Each Monday before Rudy's arrival, Bob continued to ask me, "What am I supposed to do with him?" I grew so weary of this question; I decided to talk to Rudy about it. That afternoon after Bob went to take a nap, I told Rudy privately about my frustration. He explained without hesitation, "There will come a time when he does not need to be the host. Right now, he's not there yet. He still feels like he is the host, and I am the guest." It made so much sense, but something I never considered.

After Rudy left, I began to cry. Bob had always loved being the host. And he was good at it. I remembered him at our parties, greeting guests, taking their coats, getting drinks, and making sure everyone was having a good time. I began to grasp the fact that being a real host was never going to happen again for him. Rudy understood and was kind and gentle with him.

While grateful for Rudy's explanation, I was sad for another loss Bob and I were experiencing, even if Bob seemed unaware of it.

We continued to welcome Rudy on Monday afternoons during the years Bob participated in the Friday Mind Boosters. Rudy became a witness to Bob's decline and my partner in caring for him.

Eventually, we canceled Monday with Rudy due to a change in Bob's schedule. I talked with him in advance of making the change, and he assured me he saw the common sense of our thinking. In turn, I assured him if things changed, I would contact him to resume caring for Bob. We had a big hug, and I thanked him again for all he had done for Bob — and me.

Part Three

Anger, Denial, Guilt, and Acceptance

CHAPTER 13

My Shock at Bob's Loss of Words

At the time of Bob's diagnosis, no one in the medical community, at least as far as I knew, was recommending the importance of physical exercise for a person with memory loss. Now regular exercise is as routinely suggested as socialization, a balanced diet, mental stimulation, and other activities.

Fortunately, exercise had been a part of Bob's life since he was a teenager, and although unaware of the possible benefit to his memory condition, he knew he needed to continue working out for his well-being. Riding his bicycle around the golf course every other day had been his exercise of choice since our move to Napa. However, following a minor accident a few years earlier, he felt shaky on the bike. I was on the lookout for a new exercise routine for him when I learned about an adaptive physical education class at our local community college. I suggested it to Bob and he began attending the class twice a week.

I accompanied Bob on the first visit and was impressed by the equipment in the workout room. It was scattered throughout the room, available for whatever challenge a student had.

I could see that not everyone in the class had memory challenges; some were physically challenged. It made no difference to Bob. I was grateful for his acceptance of people with disabilities. He was not always so tolerant.

He came to love the instructor. She was an engaging, athletic, middle-aged woman who was friendly to all students. At the first meeting, she put him on a stationary bike—the perfect equipment for him.

She also organized potluck parties for the group whenever there was a holiday. Bob could never remember what food he was supposed to contribute to the potluck, so I stopped by the class one day and reminded her that he and some of the others needed a written reminder about the party. She laughed at herself for assuming they could remember to bring taco chips. She assured me she would provide reminders in the future. And there were. Eventually, I shared the transportation duties with another caregiver I knew from Mind Boosters, easing the driving time for both of us. It was good for both Bob and me that he had a new social outlet and regular exercise.

This situation was not to last. The community college began to restrict the number of times a student could repeat a class. Bob was approaching that limitation. Fortunately, there was soon to be a new fitness center near our home at about the same time. We would both miss his college class group, but I knew we should join the new gym as soon as it opened. Bob was now 78, and I wanted him to learn his way around the facility before suffering more memory loss. I also wanted the staff to know him, so they could step in if he needed help.

My Shock at Bob's Loss of Words

On one occasion, as we were about to leave our new gym, I noticed that Bob did not have his cane. When I asked him where it was, he looked puzzled but had no answer. I knew he couldn't remember where he had left it. As I began searching, two staff members quickly joined in to help. One located the cane in no time. I was relieved to have their help, especially because Bob was confused and didn't seem to know where to begin looking.

The friendly helpfulness of the staff aside, the new large gym with its open spaces, high ceilings, and many exercise rooms intimidated Bob. He made it clear he didn't want to be on his own there, or at least not without me. I understood his concern. I also realized it meant giving up my original plan to drop him off to exercise while I took advantage of some alone time, as I had when he went to the college class. I told myself going with him would be a way I could get regular exercise too—something I sometimes put at the bottom of my "To Do" list.

The gym had the same kind of recumbent bike that Bob had used at the college class. I always adjusted it to his body and then signaled for him to get on the bike. Then I would get on a stationary bike in the row in front of him. In that position, I figured I could see if he left the area before I'd finished my workout.

One particular day, he seemed tired when we arrived, but I counted on the workout giving him an energy boost. The irritated look on his face whenever I turned around to check on him showed the energy boost wasn't working. I was disappointed that his spirits didn't seem to be improving but resumed peddling. When I looked back to check on him after what seemed like only a minute later, he was not there. Despite my vigilance, he had managed to escape.

When Bob didn't want to do something, he could find a way to get out of it. I was the one now who wanted him to exercise to improve his mood and counted on his unspoken agreement.

Feeling irritated that his escape shortened my workout, I got off my bike to try to locate him. Eventually, I spotted Bob sitting in a chair next to the wall between the two large exercise rooms. He was engrossed in a magazine, but as I walked toward him, he looked up with a big smile, a much different attitude than I'd seen earlier. "Would you ever do business with this guy?" he asked. He was pointing to a photo of an insurance salesman in a local throw-away magazine.

Before I could answer, I already felt a sense of relief. Not only did I see Bob's mood had changed, but he could still play one of our simple games: Showing each other a photograph of someone trying to sell some service or product, then asking if the person looked trustworthy. We always compared our answers and liked that we always agreed.

But this time, I said, "Believe it or not, we've already done business with that guy."

"What?" he asked. "How can that be?"

I explained, "You remember when we owned the condo? Well, we purchased our homeowners' insurance through his agency."

"I don't know what you mean," he said with a bit of a frown, getting up from the chair and walking toward the exit.

I pursued, as I always did, thinking if I could give him a cue that would stimulate the right neurons, he would know what I was talking about. "The condo we used to own downtown. You know, Tom lived there as our tenant." We had just seen Tom two days earlier. I was sure that it would bring a picture to mind.

Bob started shaking his head as he continued to walk. "I don't know what you mean, "condo."

Unfortunately for both of us, I rarely gave up after one attempt. I was almost compulsive about needing to prove to myself that Bob was not getting worse. I didn't think about it as a form of denial. I tried it again. "Remember the condo we bought downtown on Warren Street?"

"No, I don't," he said. He acted irritated, as if he'd lost interest.

Again, I couldn't seem to let the subject drop. "The condo on Warren Street where the two neighbors complained all the time about our renter's barking dog and everything else he did."

"Oh, now I know what you mean!" he said, looking visibly relieved. Thankful for this reaction, I asked him right away what had happened. If I hesitated, the memory was gone, lost to us both. In retrospect, I think my questioning was yet another way to reassure myself I could help Bob with his communication.

"Did you just not picture where the condo was?" I had owned a condo in the Bay Area before we were married and was pretty sure that's where his confusion came from—which condo I had meant.

"No, I didn't know what 'condo' was," he said, as we approached our car in the parking lot.

"The word 'condo' meant nothing to you?"

"That's right," he answered.

"Is that anything like when you try to find a word to tell me something and it just won't come out?" I persisted.

"Yes."

I opened the car door for him. While his concentration went to getting himself in, part of me wanted to lean up against the car itself and have a good cry. I had assumed the kind of word loss he just experienced would happen much later. Bob was only four years into the disease.

I knew that most people over 50 struggle from time to time to find a word or a name. But Bob's forgetting the meaning of a common word frightened me. It was the first time he had lost a word completely.

As I walked around to the driver's side of the car, I tried to think about how I'd be able to use this new information, this new downturn. I knew there was nothing I could do to help him. I had gradually accepted the fact that he had Alzheimer's even though he'd not received that specific diagnosis. I did realize I needed to try to stop using so many words with Bob, especially on a day when he seemed out of sorts.

Why hadn't I just let it go when he first said he didn't know what I meant by "condo"? Because that would have meant I accepted the sign of more decline. I couldn't do that yet.

CHAPTER 14

Support Group Success

Almost two years after Bob and I left our first support group, we were finally able to join a new one in Napa.

I had talked several times with Kristin, the leader of Bob's Mind Boosters group, about finding a support group. She assured me the Adult Day staff was working on putting one together. Eventually, she called to tell me they had found the resources to start a group for participants in Mind Boosters and a separate one for their caregivers. I was so pleased, and I couldn't wait to tell Bob.

When he returned home that day from his usual errands, I was waiting at the door. "Good news, Bob. They're starting a support group at the Adult Day building. You'll be in a group with the guys from Mind Boosters, and Evelyn will be the facilitator. You remember Evelyn from our interviews in Santa Rosa before we joined the first group?" I hoped he'd be enthusiastic upon learning that men he knew and liked would be in this new group and that Evelyn, not someone new, would be the facilitator.

He didn't react to my happy announcement. He had taken to refraining from acknowledging my comments, and I never knew if he was taking time to process my words or if his mind was on something else. His silences had forced me to set a new goal: try not to worry about the silences. So far, I had been only partially successful.

This time, though, he produced a question. "How soon does it start?"

"Next Thursday morning. Then every week after that."

"That's good," he said.

It wasn't much of a response, but I cherished every word and was relieved he was open to trying a group again.

We drove to the first meeting, which thankfully for us both was in the same building where Mind Boosters met on Fridays. Familiar surroundings reduced Bob's anxiety, and I was grateful he recognized where we were right away. First, we found the room where his new group would be meeting.

After a quick hello to Evelyn, I left Bob there and went on to locate my meeting. It was in a small, cramped room where I saw six middle-aged women. The facilitator/therapist, Sheila, stepped forward and introduced herself. She was younger than all of us and, when the meeting started, she readily confessed she had not done this kind of group work before but hoped we would be patient with her. I saw that she was demonstrating she wasn't afraid to show us she didn't have all the answers. I learned later being vulnerable is a sign of strength, not weakness.

The group felt right to me from the start. Sheila made everyone feel welcome, and her gentle way of talking and initiating the conversation helped me relax. As we individually told a short version of our caregiving story, it seemed almost everyone was at the same point of adjusting to our husbands' memory and cognitive problems. Every story hit me emotionally even though—or perhaps because—it matched mine: difficulty getting a diagnosis, changes in responsibility as a wife, and conflicts with our husbands as daily challenges demanded more of us.

The format was similar to my earlier group. At the start of each session, we did individual check-ins telling as much or as little as we were comfortable sharing. Sheila cautioned us not to ask questions during check-in time. I appreciated this as it was hard for me to tell about an incident if everyone offered advice or asked questions before I finished my story. A rush to provide solutions felt more invasive than helpful to me.

As I listened to the women's experiences each week, I was amazed at how many of our husbands' behaviors were similar. We were all struggling to control their difficulties with financial matters, their regular loss of everyday items, their irritation at our communication ("I don't know what you're saying," our husbands often said to us), and their confusion in general.

When I heard about the others' struggles, I could forgive myself for not doing the perfect thing in any given situation with Bob. We were all trying as hard as we could in a world we didn't understand. The loss of control over our lives seemed hard for each of us, even though we didn't talk about "loss of control" per se. My feeling was that none of us wanted to admit that maintaining a modicum of control was an essential part of our strategy for getting through each day.

Bob and I didn't talk much about what went on in our respective groups. But as the weeks went by, he began to complain that the other guys only told stories from the past. He said, "When I asked if anyone felt depressed, they acted like they didn't know what I was talking about. Then one of them told another story that had nothing to do with depression." I suggested he talk to Evelyn about his concerns when he felt comfortable doing so, but to wait until the others had left the room.

However, I decided not to wait. Bob's reluctance to speak up for himself became more frequent as his disease progressed, and I worried he might give up on the group without notice. At my next meeting, I told Sheila about Bob's concerns. She suggested I speak to Evelyn, which I did. Evelyn said Bob had not mentioned his concerns, but that she was not surprised by his comments to me. "I think Bob is one of the few guys who has been in a group before. He knows more about what kinds of topics are appropriate and may be more willing to share his feelings." Although she didn't offer a solution, I was pleased she was aware of the situation.

I relayed that conversation to Bob on the way home that day, but he didn't say much in response. I left out my regret that I couldn't change the situation for him. I did not want him to believe I could make any problematic situation better, even if I still thought I could. I wanted him to continue to try to stand up for himself. As to whether my efforts to keep him as independent as possible were for his benefit or mine, I honestly didn't know.

A few weeks later, Sheila announced at the beginning of my group meeting: The agency was going to disband the husbands' group due to limited participation. Some of the men had dropped out, and there were no new participants to take their place. I was not surprised, but I was disappointed and felt Bob would be too. When he and I talked about it at home that night, he told me Evelyn explained the same thing to his group.

"What do you think?" I asked.

"Well, it's too bad. But I am tired of hearing those guys brag about the big deals they made 10 or 20 years ago." He walked out of the kitchen before I could respond with a reassuring comment. My heart went out to him, but I didn't know what to do. Rather than follow him and try to continue the conversation, I decided to wait until after he had time to absorb the news to see if he wanted to seek individual counseling. Sometimes I tried too hard to solve problems before the timing was right.

My group of caretaking wives continued for some time. As we grew more confident and open with each other, there were few topics we didn't explore. I learned so much from others' experiences and suggestions. When I told the group about a recent trip to Florida for Bob's brother's funeral, I described how difficult it was to find a restroom for Bob in an airport as often as he now needed one. Also, I was beginning to worry he would get lost even though I stayed close by, outside the restroom. A former travel agent in our group suggested he wear pull-up Depends for any incontinence during the trip. That way, at least if he had an accident, it wouldn't be embarrassing. I thought this was a great idea and would take considerable pressure off me to always be on the lookout for a bathroom. Later that day, I told Bob about the idea." Would you be willing to try wearing Depends when we travel?"

Surprisingly, he gave me a big smile and said, "Of course. That's a great idea." I realized then how worried he must have been during our trips.

When I told the group Bob's response, they all seemed so happy for me to have this solution in place for our travels. We did try it on our next vacation, and it made a big difference in the stress I felt traveling with him.

At another meeting, one of the women told us about a non-emergency fire department phone number to call in case a loved one falls. Firefighters were available to come to your residence to assist in such situations. The phone number was not in the book, and Bob had not yet fallen, but to know where to call was calming.

We wives all had situations in common, but we also had different challenges from which I was able to learn. One woman lost track of her husband at a Fourth of July celebration. He walked away and disappeared when she wasn't looking. Although he finally returned, she had called the police and reported him missing. She added that the police encouraged her to register his name with them in their emergency database so they would have all the information if he were to go missing again. We each felt such empathy for her yet benefited from her unfortunate experience.

We were all taken aback when one participant told us her husband was getting up in the middle of the night and wandering around the house. She was awakened by the noises he made so she would hurriedly try to get him back into the safety of his bedroom. Sheila suggested we all have special safety locks installed on the doors leading to the outside. I dreaded the day my sleep might be interrupted by Bob's night wandering, yet thanks to this woman's openness, I felt more prepared to address it if it happened.

At the end of one session, Sheila asked if we would be open to focusing on a specific topic for discussion the following week instead of our free-form approach. We all nodded our heads in agreement, wondering what the subject might be. Then she cautiously said, "I think it might be helpful to talk about any problems you might be having in your sex lives since your husbands' Alzheimer's. Would you be willing to do that next time?"

"What sex?" exclaimed one of the participants. The room exploded in laughter. We all volunteered that part of our marital relationships had disappeared, and there was nothing to discuss. Sheila looked embarrassed, but we reassured her we appreciated her concerns. I had learned, at one of my first support group meetings, there were cases where the person with Alzheimer's could become sexually aggressive, and I realized Sheila was probably trying to open the door to that discussion.

After a couple of years, Adult Day decided to shift its resources to another program. The change signaled the official end of our group. Having been given plenty of time to think about what to do, we decided to continue on our own without a facilitator. We settled on meeting for breakfast at a café where we would alert the waitstaff about the purpose of our meetings and hoped they would let us stay and talk after our meal.

We met that way for years as slowly, one by one, our husbands passed away. Our shared lives during that time created a strong bond; we still get together at Christmas time to check in with each other.

In 2006, Bob and I began attending another type of support group through Mind Boosters. The agency wanted to try out a new model, one meant to combine Mind Boosters participants and their caregivers/spouses for a meal and conversation. We met once a month on Tuesday evenings at the Mind Boosters building. First, we had a potluck dinner that provided social time for everyone, especially caregivers who could get to know each other for mutual support. Afterward, we broke into two support groups: Each group then had time to talk openly without our spouses present.

The potluck dinner lasted about an hour, with caregivers doing most of the talking. There was no organized menu, but usually we ended up with a variety of salads, entrees, and desserts. Bob loved all those choices until one evening when no one brought a salad. His obsession with vegetables had been on the increase and regularly focused on salads. I was afraid if he didn't have a salad he might want to go home. When I saw how upset he was when he didn't see any salads, I approached one of the facilitators. She knew Bob well enough to know that "No salad?" was a big problem. She quietly went into their commercial kitchen and found enough lettuce and vegetable ingredients to make a salad for Bob and earned my gratitude for rescuing us both.

At the dinner table, the conversation was limited; some of the Mind Booster participants couldn't socialize and eat at the same time. I noticed that Bob's attention at the dinner was also more focused on his food. He also began to struggle in the support group meeting, now becoming one of the guys who couldn't follow the directions from the facilitator/therapist. Each evening ended with him frustrated after the group meeting.

In the months that followed, many couples did not attend regularly. Developing camaraderie became somewhat challenging. In addition, we caregivers were a mix of husbands and wives. I noticed that the husbands seemed to want concrete answers to difficult situations the group could not provide. One man wanted the caregiver group to agree with his decision to leave his wife alone in their home for a few days while he went to a conference. I found his request out of touch with his wife's condition, which I had observed at dinner. Others in the group had also seen his wife and noticed her limitations. None of us was willing to tell the man to go ahead and leave her. His frustration with our queries to him ("Could a neighbor check in on her?" "Is there anyone who could stay with her?") made him more irritated and created tension in the group.

I never heard if he left her alone or not. Bob and I eventually stopped attending the monthly get-together. In going as long as we did, I again learned from other caregivers. The issue of our loved ones asking the same question over and over (for example, "When are we having lunch?") was a regular topic of conversation. The therapist suggested that instead of repeating the answer yet again or becoming annoyed, it was usually best to ignore the question and "redirect" the person's attention to something else. "Did you see that yellow bird in the front yard this morning?" This technique was hard to learn, but I found it more effective in helping me stay patient.

Seeing other couples and hearing their stories during dinner was also helpful—everyone had unique ways of dealing with the difficulties of dementia. Also, I liked meeting the guys that Bob had made friends with at Mind Boosters.

Although his days of being part of a group were over, I was lucky my old group of wife caregivers was still meeting. Given my experiences, I was convinced the best thing a caregiver can do for herself is to find an appropriate weekly support group and make use of all the resources it provides: friendship, information, warnings, mutual care, humor, understanding, and love. We caregivers need them all.

CHAPTER 15

Disappointment Turns into Anger

It was the Fourth of July weekend, and I had awakened in a positive mood, looking forward to the day. Since Bob's memory and communication skills had diminished, our social outings had become limited, but today would be different. At breakfast, I reminded Bob that this was the day that we were meeting friends at the afternoon music concert at Veteran's Park in downtown Napa.

His only reaction was to say, "Oh?" I heard a question in his statement, but it was not what I had hoped for. Bob loved music, and live music was always a treat—but infrequent in the last couple of years. I was beginning to realize that more detail was necessary for him to track down future plans in the memory parts of his brain. I added that we were planning on meeting one of his friends from Mind Boosters and his wife at the park. They had been to this free music event before and had suggested that the four of us go together.

"Now I remember," he answered. A smile crossed his face, and I could tell he felt more confident about the plan having recalled it.

I left the kitchen and headed to my office to complete some consulting work. I watched Bob walk into the living room, hoping he would entertain himself.

In the late morning, I finished my work and knew I needed to prepare an early lunch for us so we could be at the park around noon as planned. After I chopped fresh carrots and celery, I called Bob to lunch. He made his way to the kitchen and immediately chose a carrot to munch on as I finished making the sandwiches.

Focusing on the sandwiches, I heard him cough, but I wasn't concerned. The coughing continued, and when I turned to look at him, he seemed to be struggling. I gave him a couple of firm pats on the back, and after he swallowed hard, he seemed okay to me.

"It's still stuck in my throat," he barely managed to say.

I looked at him again and said, "Just swallow hard a couple of times, and that feeling will go away."

"No, it's stuck. I have to go to the hospital."

I was sure that the carrot had bruised his throat and I tried to explain that to him. This explanation apparently made no sense. He repeated that the carrot was stuck and began to demand that I drive him to the emergency room. We were on the edge of a serious argument even after I explained that if we made the 40-minute trip to the ER, waited to see a physician, and drove back to Napa, we would no doubt miss the concert. He rarely became angry with me, but this time, I could see his anger gaining steam. He was determined to visit the ER.

My irritation escalated to anger as well. "Fine, we'll go and ruin the whole day. You'll have to explain to the nursing staff what happened. I'm not going to be the communicator this time," I yelled at him. I marched off to get my purse and keys while Bob got himself to the car with no assistance from me.

We drove in silence and walked into the ER, not speaking to each other. At the nurses' station, Bob handed his identification to a friendly man who had already opened the window. He asked, "What can we do for you today?"

I looked to Bob with an expression that said, "Okay, go ahead and tell him." He wasn't able to get a sentence started. I waited for him to answer the nurse's question, but none was forthcoming.

"He swallowed a carrot, and he thinks it's still stuck in his throat," I finally snapped at the nurse.

My angry statement didn't faze the gentle nurse. "Come on in, Mr. Jacobs, and let's take a look at you." The nurse did a brief check of his heart and vital signs and moved us into the ER department where a full examination would probably take place. He helped Bob lift himself onto the side of the bed and added, "A doctor will be with you in a few minutes."

Three hours later, the doctor pronounced him healthy and assured him that his throat was fine. Bob thanked the doctor and walked confidently out of the building. We walked to the car without any conversation.

On the drive back home, Bob eventually said, "Are we going to the concert now?"

"Oh no, we're going home. We've missed the concert because we've been at the ER all day," I said, with more than a hint of sarcasm. Bob didn't respond and continued to stare out the window. We drove in uncomfortable silence all the way home.

That evening, I began to feel guilty about my loss of patience and lack of tolerance for his worries. I had let my disappointment at missing the concert rule the day. I wasn't proud of the way I had behaved. I didn't think of myself as a mean caregiver, but that day, I qualified as one on most accounts. I vowed to work on managing my anger, even when things didn't work out as I had hoped.

CHAPTER 16

My Need for Appreciation

Almost two years after his diagnosis, Bob began to postpone a once simple routine and pleasant experience — taking a shower.

My first thought was that this personal neglect was part of the normal aging process; maybe he didn't care much about his appearance anymore. It was such a contrast to earlier years. Bob's habit always had been to dress in business casual, even though he was retired. That part of his appearance hadn't changed. He wore khaki pants with a long-sleeved button-down shirt in the summer and turtlenecks with a plaid flannel shirt and tan cords in the winter. When he went to Mind Boosters, Bob always looked ready to go to work, as he had when he went to his volunteer activities. I was pleased that his appearance still meant a lot to him.

Despite Bob's care with what he wore, I saw that his usual concern with personal grooming was fading. From the stubble on his face, I could tell he had not shaved, as he customarily did when he showered. His graying strawberry blond hair became oily and stringy after just one day and was an additional clue to me that he had not been in the shower. Even though his clothes were as clean and neat as always, his beard and dirty hair were dead giveaways that he was not attending to them. I could only conclude he was not showering often enough.

It took me a long time to figure out that Bob's infrequent showering was related to his disease. The other wives in my support group began to mention that their husbands were also avoiding the shower. We all thought it might be resistance to being told what to do. Eventually, I made the connection between the shower problem, and how the disease had affected Bob's balance—the shower was a scary place. Not only were there slippery surfaces and a raised entrance to negotiate, but also hot and cold water knobs to regulate, plus different soaps for hair and body. Furthermore, Bob would naturally shower without his glasses so that reading the shampoo and conditioner labels was confusing for him.

I found myself reminding him regularly of the need to shower. He answered my suggestions with various excuses: "I don't need to shower." "I don't have time." "It's too cold." He would usually walk away when I started my shower suggestions.

One day, in frustration at again seeing his dirty hair when he was ready to leave the house, I cruelly said, "You're beginning to look like a homeless person." Not only did my comment not affect his shower frequency, I felt ashamed I had resorted to such a negative approach. I was at the end of my rope and didn't like seeing him so unkempt. My fear was also that people might think he had no one to care for him, even though I was working hard to be a loving caregiver.

One morning after some months of this ongoing struggle, he more readily agreed to get into the shower. It was Friday, and that meant it was Mind Boosters, the most important date on his calendar each week. He never wanted to miss it and now also tried not to be late.

Bob took his clean clothes into the bathroom as I started the water to get the temperature right for him. The once easy and daily habit had become a delicate operation for us both. Our white tiled shower was open on two sides without a door, and there was that one step to be negotiated over the raised entrance. Although we had three grab bars recently installed to prevent a fall, I noticed that Bob found it difficult to use them. I reasoned that getting in and out of the shower made him nervous and that I might be able to reduce his anxiety if I stood behind him and guided him in, reminding him to hold onto the bars. The extra help seemed to reduce his hesitance. Once he was in the shower, I would usually leave the bathroom, but stay close by in the adjoining master bedroom in case he had difficulty.

After he washed with a washcloth, it became part of his routine to shout the same question to me every time before starting to wash his hair, "How much shampoo should I use?" I would go back in the bathroom and see him holding the shampoo bottle in one hand, the other hand cupped and ready for the shampoo as he looked to me for directions.

I would always respond, "Enough to equal the size of a quarter." Bob was such a visual guy; I thought the image of a quarter would stay with him. It did not. But the teacher in me would not let it go. I kept trying to make the size and shape of the coin his guideline, repeating the same instructions for each shower. He would pour an amount in the palm of his hand and look to me for approval. I would say,

"Yep, that's just about the right amount." Then he felt confident to begin washing his hair.

After the shower, Bob was able to step out onto the cotton bathmat (recommended to me by the social worker who inspected our house for safety issues), using the grab bars to help himself exit, and then dry himself without assistance.

On this Mind Boosters' morning, I was concerned that it was getting late, so I reminded him to shave. Some months earlier, he had switched from shaving with a straight edge in the shower to using his electric razor and sometimes forgot that he hadn't shaved. Now he looked irritated as if he were holding himself back from saying something.

I finally asked, "Are you upset with me?"

He said, "You're so good at doing everything, it makes me feel…" He couldn't finish the sentence.

I asked, "Does it make you feel bad?"

He hesitated and struggled to find the word he wanted. "Stupid," he said.

I was on my way out of the bathroom when I heard "stupid." It took me by surprise. Even as Bob lost the ability to do so many basic tasks, I never once thought of him as stupid and immediately wondered if I had caused him to feel that way. With my back to him and feeling both sad and angry, tears filled my eyes. My immediate thoughts were, how could a person who has trouble doing so many things, be so sensitive about someone helping him. If he were helping me, I think I would be grateful. At that moment, I felt unappreciated. Bob rarely said, "Thank you," in these situations, and I still wanted to feel some gratitude for all I tried to do for him. I collected myself, dried my face with a tissue, and turned back to face him.

"You mean when I tell you to shave, you feel like, if I just gave you more time you'd figure out what was next. Since I don't give you that time, you feel corrected?" He nodded his head.

It was a moment of great frustration for me: damned if you do and damned if you don't. I couldn't imagine not helping him, yet doing so created bad feelings between us. It was clear I didn't always handle things perfectly, but I was trying my best. And my beloved, compromised husband could not see that.

Having been with him so many years, I also knew that Bob's feeling about being corrected was a long-standing issue stemming from a childhood where most things had to be done perfectly. My family was exactly the opposite— good enough was just that. It was hard for me to remember that while his memory was failing about many everyday things, feeling corrected was a live wire that responded to the lightest touch.

Our whole lives together now demanded a balancing act I was still trying to achieve: meet time deadlines and show Bob the proper respect in giving directions and instructions. I know that I tried too hard to be efficient because I had no time for anything extra. An afternoon nap was a guilty pleasure I could only take while he was away. I couldn't stop thinking about all the work I had to do: invoices to prepare from last month's consulting work, a workshop to design, personnel policies to draft, and a myriad of household chores that Bob could no longer do for us. The list was endless.

So was my education about Alzheimer's disease. Which changes in his behavior I should watch for was a mystery, at least in those early years. When a sign did present itself,

I would first feel a sadness that more decline might be forthcoming. Second, and later, I would have a conversation with myself to try to minimize the situation so I could go on. Some people might call this denial, but it was my initial way of acknowledging every new change in him.

In my various interior conversations, I vowed to stop trying to speed things up, especially when Bob was doing personal care. The length of time for the whole bathroom routine became longer every couple of months as his need for assistance grew. Any formerly simple task for him meant I needed to build in more time. Too often, I didn't create enough, which led to my lack of patience and Bob feeling pressured.

The Bob I knew and loved was still inside there, live wires and all. I wanted to stay connected to that Bob as long as I could, and I knew it took patience and care. Some days I was short of both.

Bob made it to Mind Boosters that day, clean-shaven and neatly dressed. In a flurry, he located his car keys, wallet, and his green canvas Mind Boosters bag, full of activity papers from previous sessions. And yes, he was late.

CHAPTER 17

When Anger Gets in the Way

Three minutes into a presentation called "Compassionate Communication" for caregivers of people with dementia, I began to feel myself tighten up, especially in my shoulders and neck. It was a familiar signal to me that something was wrong.

The presenter, an attractive woman I'll call Nancy, was much younger than the majority of the audience. She was probably in her late twenties and dressed in business casual attire. It was clear she was not old enough to be a caregiver for her spouse. She told us that her grandmother had dementia when she was a child, and I assumed that this fact was to assure us that she knew what we were going through.

Nancy started her presentation by telling the audience that she wanted to make sure everyone had some general information about dementia before she addressed the subject of communication. The audience of about two dozen people were professional caregivers from private agencies or caregivers I knew from Mind Boosters or Adult Day—all of us familiar with the terminology of dementia. Did Nancy not have this necessary information about her audience? To calm my nascent anger, I took a deep breath and tried to reassure myself I didn't have to do anything. Just sit and listen.

That proved difficult. I'd heard the same unscientific grade school explanation about dementia many times, but this time was much worse, for it was much more patronizing and condescending. Nancy seemed confident her audience did not understand the difference between dementia and Alzheimer's. The first Powerpoint slide, consequently, showed the word FLOWER in large letters with the words tulips, roses, and pansies underneath it. She said dementia is like the flower, and Alzheimer's is like the rose. Why couldn't she have said, as we all knew, that Alzheimer's is one type of dementia? The irony of choosing beautiful flowers to describe these dreadful diseases of the brain must have never occurred to her.

The next slide showed an MRI (magnetic resonance imaging) scan of two brains after death, one which was healthy and one with Alzheimer's. She said, "I think this shows what's going on in the brain of a person with Alzheimer's."

I had only seen a CT (computerized tomography) scan of Bob's brain. I couldn't tell what was going on at all in the MRI she showed. My itch to speak overcame me, so I raised my hand to ask a question. When she acknowledged me, I said, "Everyone in the room has probably seen numerous CT scans of their loved one's brain but not an MRI."

Her response was supposed to be educational, but she missed my point entirely. "A CT scan is hard to read; an MRI is actually easier to read, and now they have PET (positron emission tomography) scans you can get, and they show all these colors of where there is brain activity."

Then I was especially offended because of her simplistic and misleading answer about the availability of PET scans. What she couldn't know was that I had asked for a PET scan from Bob's primary care doctor and was told Kaiser didn't have the equipment and that PET scans were still considered "experimental."

However, Bob had a PET scan as part of a research project at UC Davis, but we had to agree in advance that all tests they ran were for their research and not available to us. Still, we had spent the majority of a day going to a Veteran's Hospital in Sacramento to have the scan. The day before the trip, I had broken a bone in my foot. It had been a difficult trip on every level. The PET scan topic, therefore, was a touchy subject for me.

My internal dialog changed to silent instructions to the presenter: Do not tell me you can get a PET scan because we *can't*. I felt the adrenaline coursing through my body. I wanted to have a good argument, but I told myself again to calm down and watch.

Then the "Communication" slides began. I had taught communication skills courses for years to managers and supervisors in the workplace. I knew how hard it was to change one's communication habits, and even motivated managers struggled mightily to change theirs. Nancy read out loud the information on the slides (even though we could read them ourselves) and told us that to be a compassionate communicator one needs to be patient, an active listener, and so on. It was basically a list of good communication skills that nine out of ten people do not have. I did learn a new acronym on one slide: "pwd" referred to a "person with dementia." This acronym could be offensive to anyone caring for a person with such an illness.

Mixed in the basic list were skills needed specifically to care for such pwds: Don't correct the person when they have the facts wrong, give them time to speak, and eliminate distractions. As I well knew, and as virtually everyone else in the audience probably knew, these skills were easy to describe but difficult to do. It was likely none of us had the opportunity to learn them in advance of becoming a caregiver, and we no doubt had already developed some bad communication habits. I know I had.

Sometimes, when Bob and I were in the car, I would make the mistake of trying to tell him a story. I would forget that while he was driving, the whole outside environment was a distraction to him. He frequently interrupted me by pointing out something that struck his fancy, such as the vanity license plate on the car in front of us. There went my story.

I raised my hand again. Only one or two other people in the audience had asked any questions at that point, and I wished others would contribute what their caregiver experiences were and, of course, how it differed from the presentation. We were graduate students in the school of caring for a person with any form of dementia and were being talked to like first graders. It was insulting.

When Nancy acknowledged me, I said, "These are all good ideas, but none of us were trained to be a saint." I could tell she didn't like my comment. Someone offered that dementia is a disease of emotions and defended the list on the screen.

I was struck by this comment. I thought of dementia as a disease of the brain. No one understands why it happens, no one knows how long it will take for the person to die, but they all will die—usually a slow, painful, frustrating, and demeaning death. Yes, it's emotional for both you and your loved one because of the losses you both experience. I still couldn't convince myself to think of Bob's disease as a disease of emotions.

When Nancy referred to our loved ones as "they" throughout the presentation, further frustration built in me. She didn't know it, but there was at least one woman from Mind Boosters with her husband/caregiver in the audience. I prayed she hadn't understood the use of pwd.

To expand on her slides, Nancy explained that when a caregiver stands in front of a person with dementia, "they" will mimic the movements of the caregiver. When I volunteered I had not had that particular experience with my husband, Nancy's response was: "Well, he's not far enough along."

"Five years," I said.

"Well, the disease usually lasts 10 years. Or even 25 years," she countered.

"I hope not; he'll be 105 by then." Muffled laughs from the audience didn't help me feel better.

Nancy moved us along, "Everyone has different symptoms at different times." That was another simplistic comment I had heard many times. I was silent but fuming.

I finally calmed myself enough to know that my anger was not going to change anything or even be recognized as a common reaction for a caregiver. While wondering what the others in the audience thought, I sat quietly through the remainder of the presentation. I did promise myself I would talk about my reaction to my therapist at our next weekly meeting.

When I returned home, I walked into the living room where I saw that Bob had taken our coats out of the hall closet as if we were going somewhere. I knew I had explained to him I was going to a meeting instead of our usual Tuesday night potluck. We had had dinner at home before I left. I thought he would be all right by himself for an hour or two. Then I also saw that the dinner dishes had not been cleared from the table, and I began to piece together what might have happened.

Before I had a chance to say "Hi," and ask him how things had gone while I was away, he blurted out, "When are we going?"

Eventually, I figured it out. Bob had been waiting for me to come home so we could go to the potluck, even though I had carefully explained we were not going that night. That's why he had the coats out. Although I understood the reasons for his confusion, I was out of patience. I couldn't communicate the change in the schedule again, nor explain where I had been, nor admit I was angry, nor why. I quietly hung up the coats, cleared the table, and said, "Let's go to bed."

As exhausted as I felt, I couldn't fall asleep. I kept thinking about what was wrong with the communication class. The social workers in the room, including the presenter, were not caregivers. They would not come home to a person who had pulled out the coats and left the dirty dishes on the dinner table and had no memory of a change of plans.

When I met with my therapist, I told her about Nancy's presentation and how my emotions surfaced early in the talk and continued to the end. What had made me so angry? She helped me understand that, for whatever reason, I was probably on the edge of anger when I arrived. We then talked about ways that I could recognize the feeling and let it go. She reminded me how unhealthy it was for me to use anger as a way to feel some control in a situation. She gently told me to try to find compassion, not only for Bob but for myself. I would have to think about that. It sounded difficult.

CHAPTER 18

The Need to Help with More

arly on, Bob began to mix up details from a telephone call and in general had trouble with the phone. I would hear his frustration when I was in the kitchen, and he was on the phone in the dining room. "Slow down! You talk too fast!" he would shout at the caller.

After a couple of years, conducting any business on the phone was beyond his capabilities. He usually asked me to make the call if it was a business problem because pressing the right buttons on the phone also became difficult. When friends or relatives called, I passed the phone to him after I had started the conversation. He would mostly listen and answer common questions: "How are you, Bob?" the caller would ask.

Bob's answer was simple, "Pretty good." He would listen for a few minutes, with a blank look on his face, then hand the phone back to me without saying a word, not even "Goodbye." Assuring the caller that Bob had not hung up on them, I would finish the call and thank them for checking in on him.

I began to make most of Bob's various appointments for him. I called his doctors for advice, drove him some places, and mainly kept track of everything for him. I began to feel like Bob's assistant or mother, and no longer his wife or lover. It was hard for me to know what Bob felt.

One of the appointments he continued to arrange, by telephone, was for his haircut. He wrote the time and date in his calendar and drew a big star by the time. It was his standard symbol to indicate importance. He was still driving himself to regular meetings and appointments, so I assumed he was able to plan his departure to arrive at the barbershop on time. When he began to complain to me that Dan, the barber, was not as friendly to him as he was in the beginning, I asked what he thought the problem was. Bob was stumped. He didn't know.

He arrived home one day after his haircut and appeared upset as he told me, "Dan is mad at me."

"Why would he be mad at you?" I asked.

"I don't know. He used to be friendly, but now he barely talks to me."

That comment brought to mind that Bob used to go to my former hairstylist and stopped after he'd been late so many times that she threatened to stop cutting his hair. I was relieved, as I disliked having to explain to her he had trouble managing his calendar and assured her that I would keep an eye out to make sure he changed his ways. I wasn't successful. Since I knew this history and was neither monitoring his departure time nor managing his calendar, I asked, "Are you making it on time to your appointment?"

"Most of the time," he admitted. He didn't sound convincing.

"Maybe it would be helpful if I called Dan and made the next appointment. I'll reassure him you'll be on time as I will be driving." As I tried to sound positive, I also knew this would be another change that meant more responsibility for me. I assumed that Bob had not told Dan about his memory problems, so I didn't bring up the issue. Bob readily agreed that would be a good plan since he liked the way Dan cut his hair.

When I first called, Dan was cool and unfriendly. He seemed to soften when I explained that I knew Bob had been late for some of his appointments and that I would now be in charge of his calendar and make sure he was on time. From then on, each time I called, I always started with, "This is Cheri. I'm calling to make an appointment for Bob Jacobs." There would be silence until I asked what times were available. I don't know if the tardiness was ever discussed between them, but the tension from the past seemed still to be present. I had to build back the barber's confidence that we would be punctual.

The first time I accompanied Bob to the barbershop, I was surprised by its old-fashioned and almost charming decor. There were two barber chairs but only one barber — Dan. The walls were mint green, similar to the color of many apartments I had rented in my twenties. No attempt had been made to create the feeling of a styling salon, which had become the standard for many barbers. It could be 1958 from the appearance of the interior.

After we entered the shop, I noticed the routine they had already established. Dan would greet Bob and then take his cane in order to balance it against the wall. Bob reached for the arm of the barber chair to steady himself and then carefully lift himself into the seat.

Meanwhile, I headed for the table of magazines to relax into the world of movie gossip. I had already written the check, including the tip, to be ready for the end of the visit.

I made sure Bob and I consistently arrived on time, and the strain with Dan began to lessen. A friendliness even began to develop that made the phone calls and the visits more pleasant and comfortable. Disclosing Bob's condition to the barber seemed unnecessary now that we had a workable routine.

On one visit, after I had settled into my reading, I overheard Bob telling his story of attending the World Series between the Oakland A's and the San Francisco Giants in 1989. It was the night of the Loma Prieta earthquake in San Francisco. I remembered it well, as I was at home that evening waiting for him to call after the earthquake, to assure me he was okay. Today, I didn't mean to eavesdrop but found myself struggling to stay focused on my celebrity magazine. Then I realized that Bob was recounting his experience at a World Series game from the 1970s in Oakland between the same teams, but he was using the setting of the 1989 game in San Francisco. It was as if he had taken pieces of a jigsaw puzzle and placed them in another puzzle where nothing fit, but the pieces looked alike and were the same colors. Dan continued with his cutting and trimming, adding a comment here and there while Bob enjoyed telling two stories as one. I couldn't tell if Dan thought Bob's story was interesting.

I thought about interrupting Bob and offering the correct version, for I had always thought accuracy was important in storytelling, and it was so strange to listen to Bob tell a garbled account, but I decided to say nothing. And so it was that at Dan's barbershop, I became aware this was the kind of situation I didn't need to control.

Giving up control at appropriate times was something I had been trying in order to reduce the stress from my responsibilities. As Bob continued with no awareness of his mistakes, I knew it was far more critical for me to stay quiet and save him from possible embarrassment. No one was the wiser. Dan smiled at the story as he finished trimming the tiny hairs on Bob's neck. Bob carefully got out of the barber chair while I stood close by with the check.

"Don't forget your cane, sweetie," I reminded him. The cane was still a special challenge for both of us. We had retraced our steps many times to retrieve it from stores or wherever Bob might have placed it for safekeeping.

As we drove away, I thought about Bob's mixing the details of a story from one decade to another. It wasn't a problem I needed to deal with, yet it certainly was another sign of a deteriorating memory. Later, I wondered if being in the 1958-style barbershop had triggered something in Bob's brain to mix-up the scenes in a way that made perfect sense to him. And he seemed rather proud that he had told the story.

When we were about half-way home, Bob said, "Do you want to stop at the medical equipment store today?" He pointed out the store in the next block. I was taken aback, but I quickly put on the car's turn signal. Bob's timing could not have been better. We had gone to the store the weekend before to buy him a walker with a seat, but the store was closed. He used a standard walker from time to time, but the occupational therapist at Adult Day suggested we buy one with a collapsible seat for future needs. We had not talked about the walker since the last weekend, and I had lost track of the plan to go back another time. Six days later, it was Bob who remembered we needed to make a return visit.

As I parked the car, I turned to look at him and said, "Who has Alzheimer's?" We both laughed and shared a look that acknowledged we couldn't predict what he could remember and what he couldn't. But at least I didn't interpret his reaction as a signal that there was nothing wrong with his brain after all. The days of hoping the diagnosis was wrong were behind me.

Today, though, I was thankful Bob could still share the wonder of unexpected recall from a brain that sometimes tricked us both.

CHAPTER 19

Learning to Accept Decline

The house that we bought in the Napa Valley was built in the 1970s and had not been updated. When we remodeled the kitchen he convinced me that two stainless steel sinks and a big island in our kitchen would be a significant improvement and worth the investment. He was right.

The fact that we had two sinks made it easy for me to suggest that one would be Bob's vegetable sink where he would make our evening salad. He could work alone to wash the lettuce and then use his creativity to add whatever other ingredients he wanted. He eventually took great pride in assembling a large salad with many vegetables for most of our dinners.

We agreed that I would do the meal planning and he would be responsible for the grocery shopping. I would cook three nights during the week (to go with Bob's salad), and he would prepare meals for the other two. The weekends somehow would take care of themselves. He had learned how to make two entrees: roast chicken and meatloaf. I figured I could stand the repetition.

The most crucial division of responsibility was his agreement to do the evening cleanup: clear the table, rinse the dishes, and load the dishwasher. Loading the dishwasher was a fun puzzle project for him. He developed a specific plan for where cups, saucers, small plates, large plates, glasses, and any other dishware should be placed. Even with dinner guests, he refused help. Filling the dishwasher as full as possible was a one-person job in which he took great satisfaction.

As for me, I was delighted to cook knowing Bob would always make the kitchen look tidy. And we would regularly have clean dishes to start the next day.

This kitchen arrangement worked well for fifteen years. But when Bob started having memory difficulties, I noticed that some things in the kitchen began to change. As I started dinner preparation, I would have to remind him it was time to make a salad. "Oh, you want me to make the salad? Okay." He was agreeable but needed the reminder. I initially told myself this was not a result of his memory loss, but perhaps the result of a long day.

Eventually, Bob needed a reminder for all such kitchen tasks. In some ways, I put my prompts on a sort of automatic repeat and tried to find the compassion that my therapist, Lynne, had strongly suggested I find for such situations. She made a strong case for the power of compassion and how I needed to practice finding it for the well-being of Bob and myself. That was especially true in situations where I was tired or short of time—the perfect set-up for me to use anger to express my frustration.

As Bob's mind now drifted from such matters as making a salad, so did it move from his previous command of the perfectly loaded dishwasher and perfectly clean workspace.

More often than not, I began to find dirty dishes on the counter after he had left the kitchen as if he were all finished for the night. "Bob, are you finished loading the dishwasher?" I would ask.

"Oh, I think so. Are there more to go in?" he asked with genuine curiosity. At this point, I never noticed any irritation on his part at my reminder, though I felt exasperated at times.

As the months went by, it became commonplace for Bob to leave the kitchen with dirty dishes still on the table. Seeing him walk away from the kitchen, I would ask, "Bob, are you finished with your cleanup?"

"Yeah, why?" Now I began to hear some irritation in his response.

"Well, there are more dishes to go in the dishwasher." I tried to speak in a neutral voice with no hint of criticism.

The next time the kitchen cleanup scenario began, I felt myself getting angry even before I said anything to him. If he can't do the dishes, he should say so, I told myself. I couldn't figure out if he was giving up or his memory was failing him. Either way, I saw the whole cleanup arrangement falling apart—and falling on me.

Eventually, my anger and lack of patience buried the compassion I knew I should use. I confronted him in full interrogator mode. "If you don't want to do the cleanup anymore, you should say so. Every night the dishwasher is half-full, and I have to ask you to finish the job. Are you aware that you don't complete the job until I've called you back to finish?"

"I want to do it," he quietly answered as he walked back toward the kitchen.

"Well, what is the problem?" I asked, as my anger began to raise the volume of my voice.

He looked down at his feet and stood in silence. I waited until he found the words. "I can't remember where they go," he said without looking at me.

At that, I finally found the compassion I was supposed to keep at the ready. I put my arms around him and held him. "I'm so sorry. I didn't realize," I confessed.

Although I was inclined to ask him if he wanted to stop loading the dishwasher, my better sense said to let it go for now. We had covered enough territory.

I reassured him everything was fine and suggested walking him to the bathroom to get ready for bed. From time to time, I had begun taking the lead in getting him prepared for sleep. I always hoped it comforted him to have company and maybe helped with his end of day routine. He nodded and turned to walk to the back of the house. I followed with my hand on his shoulder, part apology and part offer of support.

He continued to help in the kitchen for a while longer, and I finally accepted that he was doing the best he could. I missed his practical assistance the more it diminished, but now the tension was gone from cleanup time. Accepting one more loss meant gaining a little peace.

CHAPTER 20

Progress with Managing Anger

I was awakened by a noise near the master bedroom door at 5:00 a.m. Bob had developed a habit of leaving his bedroom at odd times and standing in the middle of my partially open door until I would sense his presence and ask, "What's up, babe?"

This time, I knew what the interruption was probably about. Bob had gone to bed with what might have been the beginnings of a cold or an allergy attack; he didn't know which. I had a feeling, no matter what the problem was, he would want some extra care the next morning.

Now, I didn't move. I just wanted to sleep the two additional hours I'd planned on. Then he said, "I think I'm getting a cold."

"What do you want me to do?" I asked with sleepy impatience.

"Maybe take my temperature," he said.

"Bob, I'm not getting up to take your temp," I almost barked. "Go back to bed, and I'll check your temp in two hours when it's time to get up."

He walked away. My nettled response filled me with guilt, but not enough to make me get up, find the thermometer, and take his temperature. Instead, I lay there and tried to convince myself I could cope with another illness. We'd just been through a flu bug he had a month earlier and, following that, a tooth extraction that required more care and my amateur nursing. I was pretty worn out from the added-on health problems.

At 7:00 a.m. I rose, put on my robe, and found the thermometer. Bob was still in bed as instructed. I didn't need to wake him. It seemed he was waiting for me. I said, "Good morning," and showed him I had the thermometer. Without a word, he quickly opened his mouth, and I took his temp: 96.8. When I told him his temp usually ran a little low, and that's what it was today, he seemed to feel no relief.

"Let's get some breakfast in you," I said. Food had become my first-aid for many situations to bring him into the present, lift his spirits and, therefore, mine.

After eating most of his standard breakfast of yogurt mixed with grains and fruit, along with his toasted raisin bread, Bob started to tell me his concerns. "It was really scary for me last night," he said. He described the combination of things that had scared him: bad dreams, confusion about flushing the toilet, and fear of the dark. I listened to his complaints, mustering as much compassion as I could. It was so hard to understand what all of that must have felt like for him in the middle of the night.

When he finished breakfast, I followed him to his bedroom, told him I was going to run some errands, and asked if he wanted to come with me. "Oh, yeah, I'd like to go with you," he said.

This was not the answer I wanted. I was hoping to go alone so I could do the errands quickly, but I always invited him since I knew Bob loved to go anywhere in the car. I managed to hide my disappointment and my short-tempered internal question: How can you feel so bad at 5:00 a.m. that you wake up your caregiver, and then a few hours later you're ready to go for an outing?

We arrived at Walmart just in time for Bob to go to the bathroom, another test of my patience. He had begun to have ever more frequent urges to use the bathroom, even if he had gone just 15 minutes earlier. I had already learned it was no use to say, "But, Bob, you just went." Logic did not penetrate the part of his brain that initiated those bathroom signals.

We walked to the back of the store (he knew where all the restrooms were in all the stores where we shopped) only to find a plywood sign in front of the men's room which read, "Restrooms closed. Go to restroom out front of store." The former English teacher in me saw a composition problem with the sign, but when I asked a clerk, she confirmed that the restrooms were indeed outside the store. We retraced our steps to the entrance, left our empty cart where we picked it up and walked outside. Much to my surprise, there were two large porta-potties on the sidewalk. Bob noticed the one for disabled people and without a word to me, headed straight to it. Now I could see that remodeling had required the temporary restrooms, but I was only too aware of the time this misadventure had taken.

After he came out, we found another shopping cart and headed back into the store. I complained to Bob, "I have to tell you something. If I had come by myself, I would be done with the shopping, and I'd be getting in the car now instead of just starting out." The tone in my voice revealed that my impatience had taken control of my heart. Knowing his many challenges, I never wanted him to see a negative reaction on my part and, although I was surprised by my bluntness, I did not hide my frustration.

Bob had no ready response to my words or tone and finally said something like, "Oh, I didn't realize." Before his illness, Bob was the kind of guy who quickly apologized and would hug me and somehow start me laughing after a minor incident. We would have enjoyed another laugh at the wording on the plywood sign—not this time.

I did think my honest reaction helped me release some steam. I knew I was on edge and did not want to fill the day with suppressed anger. For the last few weeks, I had been struggling with my anger and was working harder to develop ways to keep it under control. Being short of sleep and feeling the stress from Bob's recent health issues, I was beginning to realize there was no shortcut to finding patience as often as I needed it.

Next, we went to the gas station. There were no pumps available, so I moved our car to the shortest line and waited for my turn. I expected that any other car would pull in behind me and wait his turn. However, the next car to arrive cut in front of me and took the pump I had been waiting for. When the driver got out and started walking toward the store to pay in advance for his gas, I stepped out of my car and shouted, "Hey! Don't leave your car there." Without responding, he continued walking to the store.

Then another gas pump became available. I went into the store and got in line to pay. He looked at me and said, "Must be having a bad day."

I answered, "My husband has Alzheimer's and every day is a really hard day."

As he paid he said, "Yeah, I know my grandmother has Alzheimer's."

"I bet you don't live with her," I said as I paid and then stormed out the door behind him.

He turned toward me and said, "You should take it a little easy."

That was the wrong approach with me that day. Giving vent to all my pent-up anger, I said, "I've put up with crap from men in business for years, and I'm sick of it." I realized that I wasn't making much sense. I was making this stranger the object of my anger, rather than directing it at Bob.

He tried to explain that he didn't notice my car at first.

I was not mollified and asked, "Are you in business?"

"Yes," he answered. After a pause, he said, "Well, I'm sorry about that. I mostly work with women, and I have many women in my family." I wasn't sure what his point was about women, but I was aware he was trying to apologize in a clumsy way.

I said, "You're lucky. You probably have a better life."

"Yes," he said, "I am lucky."

Our back and forth seemed to finally come to an end. I became aware of how much anger had built up in me. I knew it wasn't good for me. Without much thought, I started to walk toward his car, and the tears started to stream down my cheeks. I managed to say, "I'm sorry. I really am having a bad day. I can't take it out on my husband, so I took it out on you."

He looked at me, waited a moment, and then apologized. We walked toward each other and had a light hug. I was surprised but felt like something important had just happened. As I walked back to the car, I was able to take a deep breath and wipe the tears from my face. On purpose, I had not looked at Bob during the altercation. I concentrated on getting the tank filled. When I finished and got in the car, I still didn't know what to say to Bob and didn't know what he'd seen. I didn't want to tell him what I had said about Alzheimer's.

Bob simply asked, "What happened there?" It turned out, he had watched the whole episode, but he probably didn't understand anything about the shouting match.

I said, "Let me pull out of here first, and I'll tell you." Another car was behind me. Getting out was almost as difficult as getting in, except this time, I had patience. The other driver backed up, let me pass and then gave me a friendly wave as she pulled forward.

Back on the road, I said to Bob, "I was rude to that guy. I decided to apologize to him and then he apologized to me."

"Oh," he said. I knew it probably made no sense to him, and he was perhaps unaware I had been so angry.

As I drove us home, I felt ashamed of how my anger had escalated. I was beginning to see how expressing my anger made me feel more in charge, but it was short-lived and created a false sense of power. My therapist had warned me that if turning to anger became a habit, it would not be good for me. She talked about the negative effects anger creates in body chemistry and how it can become addictive. If I continued to use anger in this way, she cautioned, the opportunities to grow from my caregiving challenges would be lost.

I was surprised at how much courage it took to apologize. I felt vulnerable not knowing what his reaction might be. I hoped this would be an experience I would remember in the future, even when I wanted to stay angry and let the whole world know why.

Part Four

The Unexpected
Losses

CHAPTER 21

Social Occasions
Bring on New Difficulties

Bob completely lost his sense of taste when he first started to take the drug Aricept. Waiting a few days to see if his body would become accustomed to the drug did not work. There was precious little I could cook that had any taste to him at all. In desperation, I called the nurse practitioner on the Alzheimer's Disease Center staff and told her about the situation. She recommended I reduce the dosage and assured me their research indicated the smaller dose would be effective.

Within days of making the change, Bob's ability to taste returned, and he could enjoy food as he always had. He returned to eating two breakfasts, one before his morning exercise and one afterward.

Bob's appetite often attracted attention. Early in our marriage, we visited my 80-year-old mother in Washington State. She was still getting to know Bob's quirks and idiosyncrasies and was astonished at his ability to consume so many calories and always stay slim, a fate that often eluded both her and me. Bob, however, would eat his second breakfast as if he were home and had just finished his bike ride. One morning, as my mother watched this eating anomaly, she blurted out, "My God, that man eats a lot." I laughed at her frankness, while Bob smiled and continued to eat. He had endured this observation many times from friends and family and never let it diminish his appetite.

As Bob struggled with memory loss and the progression of his disease, eating became an even more important part of his day, yet physically more challenging. Although he looked forward to meals, he had developed a tremor in his right hand which made handling a fork difficult. Working his way through a meal took longer. The tremor, we learned from his doctor, was not related to Alzheimer's but was an "intention tremor," meaning it was activated when Bob moved his hand intentionally.

A more vexing problem, indeed related to Alzheimer's, was that Bob began to eat food meant for other people. The first time this happened — the other person was me.

We were at a fundraising event in the fall of 2007 for a local nonprofit organization. I had served on the Board of Directors for many years. The annual fundraiser was something Bob and I had attended before and enjoyed. It was a dress-up affair at a country club. Bob especially enjoyed the varied and delicious food.

When we received the invitation to the event, I recalled advice from a high school friend of Bob's. She had learned of his Alzheimer's and called me from time to time to offer support and encouragement. The one piece of advice she always repeated was, "When my husband had Alzheimer's, I took him everywhere." She encouraged me to do the same and added that it kept their relationship close, even during the last years of his disease.

I told him about the event, he said, "Oh, that sounds good." On the night of the event, I helped him get dressed in a suit and tie, a task that now took both of us. Fortunately for me, Bob was now more patient with my assistance.

Upon arrival, we made our way past the silent auction items and the crowd at the entrance to the dining area. I saw my friend Judy, who was also on the Board, and guided Bob to her table. She introduced us to her mother, visiting from Florida. While Judy and I chatted briefly, Bob made a connection with her mother right away by telling her that his parents had retired in the Tampa area. Then, out of the blue, he said, "Would you like me to go to the bar and get you a real drink?" (Only wine was available at the table.)

Her face came alive with a big smile as she said, "Stoli on the rocks with a twist, please." I loved seeing Bob's old charm at work and gladly recognized he still had those social skills at the ready, at least tonight.

The next year, the fundraising event was held at the same location, which I thought would make it familiar to Bob. Upon entering the building, the size of the crowd seemed to cause him some anxiety. I hoped for the best and sought out our table.

After the first two courses had been served, and the silent auction concluded, people began to visit each other's tables. I noticed the waitstaff starting to deliver desserts on individual white plates filled with a variety of beautiful chocolate bonbons, truffles, and mini brownies. Our waiter placed my dessert in front of me, but before I could taste it, I felt a tap on my shoulder. I turned around to find a colleague from our Board whom I hadn't seen in some time. I jumped up to give her a friendly hug and then quickly introduced her to Bob, whose attention was more focused on his dessert than on meeting a stranger.

When I finished talking, I sat back down to enjoy my chocolates. My dessert plate was empty. So was Bob's.

I turned to Bob and quietly asked, "What happened to my dessert?" His face was blank. I continued, "Well, what happened to it?" He said he didn't know.

By now, I could feel the other people at the table watching us. I didn't want to make a scene, so I dropped the subject and tried to let it go. But inside, I felt like a petulant child who was being punished by not getting the sweets she had been promised. I considered Bob might be teasing me, but it had been a long time since he had been able to pull off this kind of a stunt.

In the car on the way home, I asked again, "Bob, I want to check in with you. Did you eat my dessert?"

He had been quiet since leaving the country club; I knew this kind of outing was exhausting to him. I didn't know if he would answer. But finally, he said, "I don't know what you're talking about."

End of the conversation, at least for that night.

Over the next few days, I thought more about that evening. I wondered if I should continue to take Bob to social affairs where appropriate behavior was expected. Not only had I been embarrassed by the empty plate scene, but I also realized some part of me was still angry. Those chocolates were my reward—my just desserts—for being on caregiver duty while everyone else was having a carefree evening. Yes, I felt sorry for myself. And yes, I worried that this was another step in Bob's decline.

By then, I had been told that once a symptom in dementia starts, it doesn't usually go away. It progresses. But I hadn't totally accepted that as fact.

So I was shocked when Bob again took some food not meant for him a few months later. We were at a memorial service for the husband of a woman from my Alzheimer's support group. Following the service, we gathered for the reception at an outdoor patio. Food was served buffet style. After I found a place for Bob to sit with friends, I made my way to the buffet table to prepare a plate for him, delivered his meal, then returned to the buffet to make a plate for myself. When I returned to the table, there wasn't room for me, so I chose a seat close by keeping one eye on Bob.

When I finished eating, I went to check on him. He had finished his meal, including some cookies I had included on his tray, but now he was consuming a partially eaten brownie from a plate that someone had left in the middle of the table.

I realized he was in his own world, with no sense of whose plate belonged to whom. This time, although I felt sorry for him—a common emotion for me those days—I was angry too for his being out of control. In a kind of silent fury, I immediately cleaned up all the other leftovers so he would have no other inappropriate food to eat. I then left the area without talking to him.

A few minutes later, I went to another table filled with the family of the deceased. Then I saw that Bob had moved to sit at that table. To my surprise, he was eating cookies from a big plate from which the family's children (all with head colds) had eaten. He wasn't talking to anyone; he was eating cookie after cookie, much like a hungry, homeless man who had come upon free food.

Appalled at his behavior, yet hoping nobody else was paying attention, I leaned down and whispered to him that I thought it was time for us to leave. He followed me willingly, again as if nothing were out of the ordinary.

Feeling embarrassed by Bob's behavior was an experience I never expected nor wanted. I always admired parents of developmentally disabled children who treated their children with care and respect. I now wondered if I could do the same. I feared that Bob was fast becoming a person whom people would stare at and be uncomfortable around. If I wanted others to accept him, I had to first accept his behavior with my whole heart.

His new eating compulsion of grabbing anything he could, or at least any foods he especially liked (sometimes sweets, sometimes special items from an hors d'oeuvres table), was one of the first public behaviors I would have to come to terms with.

At the next meeting of my support group, I talked about the eating situation and also covered the topic with my therapist. They all helped me realize that social events take enormous amounts of energy from a brain with Alzheimer's. Even though Bob might do well at the beginning of a social event, as he did at the first fundraiser, his cognitive processes might weaken as his energy decreased.

I then made an important decision. I would still try to take him everywhere with me, but I needed to plan for the decline I now knew would come as fatigue took its toll. I vowed to try to anticipate his drop in energy before he regressed to socially inappropriate behavior. Also, at home, I would make sure I didn't leave the table before I was able to enjoy my dessert.

Continuing to take Bob with me to social outings seemed like a tall order, but I wanted to try. The alternative was to go alone and give up on the idea that our being together was still the best way forward for both of us.

CHAPTER 22

My Panic When He Disappears

Purchasing a car was one of the many unexpected projects I had to take on during Bob's illness. Our 1993 Volvo needed replacing before an expensive repair was required. Buying a car without his being able to test-drive it at least, seemed unfair to him and guilt-producing for me. Of course, I would be the only driver, but his acceptance of the car was important to me. And making significant dollar decisions was something we had always done together.

Luckily, our friend Judy had decided to sell her 2005 Honda Accord in 2007. I knew she took good care of her car and had it maintained regularly. I had owned a Honda Civic in the 1970s and had confidence that Hondas were well made. It was a relief not to have to bargain with an auto dealer.

Nonetheless, I had done proper internet research on this Honda model. In my poking around for information, I learned that Hondas are the most widely stolen cars in the country: all models, all sizes, all years. The parts are interchangeable and are easily resold through black markets.

This unsettling news did not distract me from the decision to buy the car. I did promise myself I would never leave it unlocked and would always set the alarm. "Safety First" would be our motto—just like many other parts of our lives these days.

The last step before making Judy an offer for the car would be to do a test drive. I wanted to be sure it could accelerate quickly on a freeway entrance. We went to her house to look over the car and make sure it was what we wanted.

I frequently asked Bob to sit in the back seat of the car to reduce his anxiety. I had learned at Adult Day that he was at the stage where his spatial awareness was declining. He would shout at me that I was too close to the curb and scare me when we were in no danger. This day, though, I asked him to sit in the passenger seat beside me. He was happy to sit in the front.

The Honda performed perfectly. Upon our return to Judy's, I said, "I think we should buy it." Bob agreed, but I could see a kind of sadness on his face. It was undoubtedly the first time he had bought a car without driving it.

It was fun for me to have an almost new car to drive. The more we drove around town in it, the more vocal Bob was about what a good car it was. Whenever we parked, I would explain to him it was necessary to lock the car and why. I knew not to give him too much information, but I wanted the message to stick in his brain that we couldn't just walk away when we were leaving the car. He seemed to understand my concern.

In the next few months, Bob's energy level and walking ability continued to decline. Although he always wanted to go with me to run errands, sometimes he preferred to stay in the car and wait while I ran into the bank or drug store. The grocery store was different. He liked going in and seeing all the items in Trader Joe's, but sometimes he struggled to determine if he had the energy to go with me. He never liked the Whole Foods store next to Trader Joe's. Something about it was confusing to him. Regardless of how many times he went there with me, he seemed overwhelmed.

One particular day when I was going to visit both stores, I drove into a parking space by the sidewalk so he would have people to watch and said, "I'm going to Whole Foods first. Do you want to go with me, Bob?"

A long pause followed by, "No, I'll stay here."

"Okay," I said. "But remember, I'm not going to lock you in." I feared that I would cause him anxiety if he tried to get out and couldn't remember how to unlock the doors from the inside. "You really must stay in the car until I get back."

"Oh, I know," he reassured me.

Off I went to Whole Foods, only a few steps away, to buy just a few items. I finished my shopping in less than 15 minutes. As I exited from the store, I saw that no one was in the car. I felt an adrenaline rush. What could have attracted Bob enough to get him out of the car? Was he wandering around the parking lot running the risk of being hit by a car? Had he gone into a store to use the restroom? How was I going to find him?

Just as I reached the car, I saw Bob coming out of Trader Joe's talking casually with an old friend from our neighborhood. They were chatting and walking along like everything was right with the world. I greeted our friend, then turned to Bob and snapped, "What are you doing? I thought you were staying in the car." Before he had a chance to answer, I noticed he was carrying a bunch of bananas in a small plastic bag from the store. I hopefully asked, "Did you pay for those bananas?"

He looked at the bananas and said, "Yes." I knew he hadn't. He never carried cash or credit cards anymore, so he would not have been able to make a purchase regardless of what he had picked up.

In an apparent attempt to lighten the situation, our friend started to laugh. He knew Bob had Alzheimer's but had not seen him in a long time to witness his decline. I had the good sense not to pursue my interrogation. At that point I told the friend we probably needed to go back into the store and pay for the fruit.

We returned to the car, but I could hardly speak to Bob. I was still so full of adrenaline from the fear I felt when I realized he was missing. I again told him that he had left the car unlocked and exposed it to possible theft. I focused on the car, but I was more upset about not knowing where he was. I knew he was unable to assess any kind of danger on his own. He quickly said, "I'm sorry." I was aware it was just to appease me. It was becoming a familiar scene with us. I was frantic and angry while he was calm as a child.

Later, I had to face the fact that I couldn't leave him alone in the car and expect that he would stay there. If he continued to want to accompany me on these shopping trips but not stay with me, how could I keep him safe?

CHAPTER 23

Sundowning Challenges

I have always been a talker. I get ideas while I'm talking. For many years, I did problem-solving by talking with others in business situations. So when I started my independent consulting practice, my biggest concern was that I did not have other human resources staff to talk with. After promising myself that I would not hire an employee, but work solely on my own, how would I get ideas if I couldn't talk to anyone?

The answer turned out to be Bob. He had no consulting experience, no human resources experience, and was retired, but he was perfect for me. After all his years as a sales manager, training and listening to his sales agents to help them be successful, he was a good listener. He had learned early in our relationship that when I talked about work, I didn't always want suggestions; I just needed to talk something out. Besides, he and I had a long history of talking about everything. Nothing was too minor to discuss.

Even after Bob's Alzheimer's diagnosis, I continued to talk to him about everything, from our cat's hunting successes brought through the pet door, to how I might be able to change the burned-out light bulb in the ceiling of the garage. As with our first conversations years earlier, he willingly listened. I always felt that even with this disease, if we could talk about a problem, I could find an answer.

My impulse extended to my support group. When others asked for a suggestion about how to deal with a new problem or behavior from a husband, I usually offered, "How about talking with him about it?" I was a firm believer that talking through a problem meant you were halfway to a solution.

Then my turn came to face the loss of Bob's ability to talk with his usual fluency. I knew that loss of communication was a common effect of Alzheimer's, but I lived with the hope (or denial) it wouldn't happen to Bob. But then it did.

About six years into the disease, he began to suffer distress brought on by what is known as "sundowning." As the sun starts setting and the light of the day fades, people with Alzheimer's commonly have unpleasant mood changes, including confusion, anxiety, and even aggression. Bob's most common reaction was to become anxious. He had always been acutely and painfully aware of each change in his mental or physical decline from the disease and would sometimes even announce he couldn't do one thing or another anymore. With the advent of sundowning, Bob began to appear nervous early in the evening. He looked like someone who dreaded facing the next hours and would walk around the house aimlessly.

As I saw his anxiety increase, mostly by noticing his restlessness, I began to dread the evening. I would softly say, "What's up, sweetie?" hoping my question would distract him and maybe prompt him to talk about something that happened during the day. More often than not, his response was limited. I tried hard not to press him for an explanation. My experience with him in our early married life taught me that he didn't like to be pressed to give information until he was ready to share.

Increasingly, Bob's body language informed me more than his words. He began to avoid eye contact with me during those times and then would say, "I'm anxious." I wasn't surprised by his answer. We had already seen his primary care doctor, and she had prescribed Ativan, which was supposed to have a calming effect on his anxiety. It helped but was meant to be for a particular situation, on an as-needed basis, not as a daily medication. Plus, it didn't have an immediate effect; usually, it took between 30 and 60 minutes to reduce anxious feelings. My ability to time the dose was critical. I needed to react to the first signs of anxiety. Sometimes I didn't notice the beginning or was busy doing something else, so I didn't give him the Ativan early enough. Other times it didn't seem to have any effect, no matter what time I gave it to him. I learned from others in my support group that his reactions, or non-reactions, were typical in trying to manage the inevitable anxiety that comes with Alzheimer's.

One evening, I had given Bob the Ativan early and then tucked him in for the night, but he got back out of bed after a few minutes. I was in the kitchen finishing up from dinner and looking forward to some quiet time by myself. I heard him enter the room and turned to ask if he was all right. Before I could utter a word, he said, "I'm so anxious."

"Do you know why?" I went into inquiry mode, not knowing what else to say.

"I had a bad dream." He paused, trying to find more words.

A bad dream? I was confused. He certainly had not been asleep yet.

"I'm afraid I'm going to have that same dream tonight," he managed to explain. I was surprised at this. I thought his short-term memory loss would have prevented him from even remembering a dream from the night before. Once again, I felt the unpredictable twists and turns of Alzheimer's changes, which left us both with less and less control over our lives.

I quietly walked him back to his bedroom and helped him back into bed. The Mozart CD he loved was still playing from the time I had put him to bed earlier. The room felt cozy to me, the low light of the small lamp from his childhood on a table in the corner. This light, or the lamp itself, sometimes helped Bob adjust to the loss of sunlight.

After he settled under the blankets, I sat next to him and gently asked about the dream. As I pieced together his description, it seemed the dream took place in his old business office where he was responsible for the sales production of many agents. While he didn't say he felt the pressure for his agency to reach specific sales targets, I thought it might have been that aspect of the dream that troubled him. He had lived with corporate pressure to achieve sales goals his whole career. He went on to describe other concerns too. Due to my fatigue, I didn't try to get more details. Instead, I went into my customary "fix-it" mode. "Why don't you try meditating?" "Couldn't you try that guided relaxation CD?"

At some point, he interrupted me and blurted out, "I'm afraid of the dark!"

It occurred to me that this exclamation might contain the kernel of truth that had eluded both of us for some time. It was amazing to me that Bob could conclude his anxiety came from fear. However, his announcement frightened me too. I tried not to panic, although my heart went out to him like it would to a small child. He was too old, though, for the comfort of a stuffed animal or a bedtime story.

Then I made the mistake of thinking I could talk him through the fear. Perhaps it might help if he understood "sundowning." I started to describe that the sun had set and created a change in the light because the days were growing shorter. He looked at me in bewilderment. Now it was time for me to face a question I never wanted to ask. "Do you expect that I'll be able to fix these things when you bring them up?"

"No," he said softly.

I sat there for a long time. While trying to think about what to say or do next, I reached for his hand, a gesture that usually comforted him. Finally, I asked, "If I just listen and care would that be enough?"

"Yes," he said with a small smile. "Let's make a pact. That's it—listen and care."

I smiled back and gently kissed him. Then I left the room before my emotions overwhelmed me. I loved Bob for being able to state such a simple truth: listen and care. Even if he was ready for this change in our relationship, I wasn't sure I was. To give up talking to him and offering ideas for help, to give up our long-lasting verbal connection, meant another significant and unavoidable loss. The sun was indeed going down.

As I tried to be grateful that Bob could still tell me what he needed, I also recalled my therapist's advice about the need for compassion. Showing him compassion by listening was probably the best medicine I could provide.

CHAPTER 24

The End of Dining Out

Bob and I had lived in the San Francisco Bay Area in the 1970s and had fond memories of our experiences in that lovely Mediterranean climate. Despite calling Napa home since 1986, I continued having my dental work done in Oakland. When Bob became ill, he accompanied me to appointments; we made an outing of the day.

One day, after seeing my hygienist, we decided to have our typical light dinner before heading home. We settled on Barney's Gourmet Hamburgers, a favorite haunt from earlier days. I parked the car as close as I could to the restaurant since Bob's walking ability had deteriorated. Even with the cane, the curbs and uneven sidewalks were difficult for him.

The choice of where to eat had become more straightforward in recent years. As Bob's ability to manage newness and complexity decreased, we began to choose familiar places, including restaurants. Familiarity with the menu and with the location of the restrooms was critical to our having a relaxing meal. Barney's fit the criteria.

We arrived early before the dinner crowd and were seated quickly. As we looked at the menu, I recalled to Bob that he liked the Greek salad. "That's what I'll have," he said and got up from his seat. I knew he was headed to the restroom and was not surprised when he left the table. This need to frequently visit a bathroom had become a regular part of his routine, especially when we were away from home.

Also, Bob had experienced a couple of urinary accidents. After the last one, he announced to me that he was going to a restroom at the first urge he felt. And he did. As disruptive as these many restroom requests were (especially when we were on the freeway), I was glad he was committed to managing the problem himself. Knowing that incontinence was part of the progression of Alzheimer's was one thing. It was another thing not to know when to expect it nor how the incontinence might progress.

I certainly did not anticipate the anxiety that went with the urges Bob struggled with daily, but I had begun to face the fact that we were already in the more severe throes of Bob's overall decline. For these reasons alone, I tried hard to accept the frequent bladder breaks with patience instead of criticism. "You just went to the bathroom at the dentist's, for crying out loud," is a sentence I would try to say only to myself.

Today at Barney's, I ordered our meal and watched the clock while waiting for Bob to return. Clock-watching had become a nervous habit: monitoring the amount of time he was in a public restroom created unwelcome tension for me. I feared he wouldn't remember where he was when he came out or wouldn't be able to find me. I usually didn't worry at Barney's; he knew the restaurant layout, and there was only one unisex restroom.

This time, Bob returned to the table in just a few minutes. I asked, "Everything all right?"

"Yeah," he said, "I couldn't go." He seemed irritated and glum. The food had arrived, and we started to eat. He took a couple of bites of his salad but again got up to leave the table in a few minutes.

"Where are you going now?" I asked, unable to hide my irritation. He either didn't hear me or was too focused on his task. He walked away. This time, he was gone for a considerable amount of time and returned just as I was ready to investigate what might have happened.

As soon as he returned, I asked, "Are you okay? You've been gone so long." He sat down, scowling, and started eating without responding. I was concerned to the point that I described to him how long he had been gone and that I was worried.

Then he angrily, if reluctantly explained, "I had trouble in the bathroom."

"What do you mean 'trouble'?" I asked.

He explained as best he could that someone came in and started yelling at him. I began to realize, that with a unisex bathroom, he may have forgotten to lock the door, and someone had entered thinking it was empty. I described this possibility. He said, "Yes, I think that's what happened." He was so confused and agitated, however, that I realized he couldn't clearly remember the details of his previous bathroom trips.

Then I suggested, "I'll go back with you and stand outside the door, okay?" He agreed. We left our food and walked to the restroom.

I went into the small bathroom with him, locked the door, and stood guard in case someone started knocking to get in. He finally gave up trying to relieve himself, but he looked angry and didn't look at me.

We walked back to the table where I quickly resumed eating my hamburger before it cooled off even more. Bob tried eating his salad but mostly picked at it as if he weren't hungry. It was unusual for the salad king. We finished the meal in silence.

I felt like one of the couples we used to observe in our early dating years who would be out to dinner together but then never talked to each other. We used to wonder if that would happen to us. Now it had. But it felt more as if I were on a blind date. I didn't know what to say to this man. He didn't seem to want to talk. So we sat in silence, eating but not tasting the food. I wondered if this was the end of our dining out.

As we left Barney's, I made myself feel somewhat better by putting my right arm through his left arm as we walked. Bob still wanted to be the gentleman, placing himself next to the street. Touch was so essential to us both. We still had that, and I needed to remember it. With his cane in his right hand, we slowly and silently made our way to the car. I drove us home again in silence. I was by now so sad I couldn't even think about what I should do next to try to make the situation better.

A few days later, I concluded all I could do was make sure there wasn't something physically wrong with Bob that caused such frequent urinary urges. Something created that anxiety, and obviously, it tapped my impatience. This was not a dynamic I wanted to continue.

I made an appointment with Bob's primary care doctor who referred us to the urologist we had seen some months earlier. That preliminary exam had been inconclusive. Now it was time for more extensive testing. Before the second urology visit, I think both Bob and I were unable to keep our expectations in line. I was hoping Western medicine could fix whatever was wrong. After a grueling procedure (filling Bob's bladder with as much liquid as he could stand, while he lay half-naked on a table, then measuring the flow and ability of his bladder to empty) the urologist said nothing.

Finally, he offered, "There's nothing wrong with his urinary system. It's the CNS." Then without waiting for a question or acknowledgment from me, he snapped off his gloves and turned to walk out the door.

I had grown accustomed to doctors speaking to me as if Bob were not in the room. They seemed to assume he was incapable of any communication. Other caregivers in my support group had frequently experienced the same thing at doctor visits. We all knew our loved ones usually could not quickly process complicated medical explanations. Nonetheless, it was hard to watch Bob be excluded from learning about the test results. In a sense, I felt ignored too, as the urologist offered such a brief explanation and did not explain what CNS meant.

The appointment suddenly over, Bob looked at me for an explanation. I said, "Let's get you dressed and get out of here." I was close to tears and just wanted to protect Bob from any further embarrassment.

As I helped him put on his clothes, I kept running the letters CNS through my memory of dementia-related vocabulary. All of a sudden, it came to me. CNS is the Central

Nervous System. The impersonal doctor used a detached way of saying Bob's brain could not give appropriate signals to his bladder.

On the way home, I decided to tell Bob that Alzheimer's was causing the problem. In the car, I reached for his hand to try to console him. I knew we were both disappointed. I never thought I'd want to hear that surgery was an option until it wasn't. The problem again was his brain.

What Bob and I learned that day, by default, was that there was nothing doctors could do. Again, we were left to our own devices to face the increasing effects of dementia. I realized Bob was trying to adjust by adding frequent trips to the bathroom. I loved him and wanted to help however I could, and it was my responsibility to manage my frustrations. That was what my brain needed to remember.

CHAPTER 25

We Learn to Accept Leaving Mind Boosters

Late in 2007, after more than four years of regular attendance at the weekly Mind Boosters gatherings, Bob began to come home on Friday afternoon out of sorts. When I asked how his day had gone, he would tell me the staff at Mind Boosters was doing something wrong. Mostly, his complaints had to do with instructions for activities. To him, the directions weren't clear and his questions not answered. He was annoyed.

I wondered if the staff was losing patience with him. I suggested he sit next to someone who understood what to do so he could hitchhike on that person's understanding. I also tried several other recommendations, none of which Bob thought would work.

Finally, after some weeks of seeing him down in the dumps after Mind Boosters, I said, "Would you like me to talk to one of the managers? I don't know what might come of it, but if that would help, I'm glad to make an appointment."

He smiled and said, "That would be great." Things seemed brighter for both of us just knowing that we had a plan.

I made the appointment and a few days later met in the administration office with the program manager and the Mind Boosters facilitator. They both listened carefully to my recitation of Bob's dissatisfactions. I was counting on them to acknowledge Bob's difficulties and then offer some changes that could be made to reduce his frustrations.

Instead, the manager said, "The problem, Cheri, is that Bob can no longer understand the directions and therefore isn't able to participate fully in the activities." The facilitator agreed, adding they had been concerned about him and were about to contact me when I called them.

As they spoke, my head started swimming. Somehow, despite what I considered my acceptance of Bob's illness, it never occurred to me that the problem at Mind Boosters was his lack of comprehension. I was so unprepared to hear the women's explanation that, after they stopped talking, I couldn't help but start to cry. A few excruciating minutes passed. Then I realized that they were waiting patiently for me to collect myself.

"Does that mean he's so incapable now that you can't have him in the Mind Boosters?" I asked, stating my worst fear.

"No, he can certainly stay in Mind Boosters for a while, but it probably is time for the two of you to talk about what the next step might be for him." I knew that the next step reference meant the day program on the other side of the building. It was provided by the same organization but was designed for adults with chronic illnesses and more advanced dementia.

The conversation moved on to the subject of the difficulties most participants had in leaving Mind Boosters and joining the day program. Because both programs sometimes had joint activities, participants in Mind Boosters were aware of the difference between the two groups. The Mind Boosters participants considered the day program (Adult Day) to be for people who were "really bad off," as they would say. Bob had made similar comments to me when he first started Mind Boosters, so I knew how distressed he would be to hear he needed to be in that program. For both of us, the move would mean accepting further decline. I already knew how disappointed I was.

After thanking the two managers for their time and saying I would be back in touch soon, I walked to the car in a bit of a daze. I began to review the number of changes in our daily lives that leaving Mind Boosters would bring. A crucial change for me involved time.

Adult Day met every day, except weekends; Mind Boosters met only on Fridays. Because Bob had stopped driving, I took him to and from Mind Boosters every other Friday, thanks to ride-sharing with another participant. I told myself not to think too far ahead, but I could already see more of my hours eaten up by being a chauffeur—if, that is, Bob agreed to go to the new program.

That night, as gently as I could, I told Bob about the outcome of the meeting. We had dinner and then went to our usual conversation place, the living room. I sat close to next him and reached for his hand. I conveyed to him what happened. "The manager told me you're having difficulty understanding the instructions, and that's why you're so frustrated. I'm afraid that it's the Alzheimer's, sweetie," I said, gingerly. Although we had always been open about the symptoms he was experiencing, acknowledging that Alzheimer's was now interfering more in his intellectual abilities was bound to be upsetting.

Bob nodded. I waited to let the news sink in before I started in on the next step I had in mind. I still didn't feel confident that the managers had totally understood what was going on with Bob. Their easy answer of moving him to Adult Day made me want another opinion about what was best for Bob at this stage of his illness. When I was sure he was not going to ask me any questions, I took his silence as a signal to continue. "I think it might be a good idea for us to meet with Kristin. She is a consultant now and knows of all the dementia programs in the North Bay."

"You mean Kristin might be able to help us?" His mood brightened at just the suggestion of talking with her. Kristin managed Mind Boosters in Bob's early days there; he developed trust and confidence in her, and I counted on him remembering that.

"I'll give her a call and see if she can meet with us. Okay?"

"Sounds good to me," Bob said, as he rose from the couch to get ready for bed. His spirits were much better; I worried that I inadvertently had given him hope he would be able to stay in Mind Boosters.

I called Kristin the next day and set an appointment for the following weekend. She offered to come to our house for the meeting, which was best for us. Meanwhile, knowing he would see her soon, Bob went to Mind Boosters as usual that Friday and seemed calmer than he had for some time.

On Saturday, before Kristin arrived, I asked Bob if he wanted to sit in on the meeting. He assured me he did. I alerted him to the fact that Kristin may want to talk with me alone at some point. When she arrived, Bob was at the front door with me to greet her and gave her a warm hug. We moved to the living room and sat down. She started a conversation with him about how he was, and they chatted easily for a few minutes. Then she said, "Bob, I think Cheri and I should talk a bit first and then we'll have you rejoin us, okay?"

He was agreeable. "Sure, just let me know."

With Bob out of the room, I recounted my meeting with the Mind Boosters staff and went into more detail about the complaints Bob had been having. Kristin asked me a couple of questions and then said, "It sounds like he's ready for Adult Day, Cheri. You know my dad was in Adult Day too, and I know he liked it."

It was not the answer I was hoping for.

"He will be happier there," she continued, "as he'll feel accomplishment again when he participates in the activities, which it seems he hasn't had for some time."

"Really?" I still thought there might be another option.

She continued, "There isn't another program in Napa County for him at this stage. I know it's hard to accept as it does mean his disease is progressing. Do you want to explain this to him, or would you like me to?" I said I thought I could handle it.

I went to get Bob from the other room to join us. His spirits seemed okay, and he appeared interested in what would happen next. I started to describe to him what Kristin had said, but it wasn't coming out right. I didn't want to make him confused or upset, so I turned to her after all. "Kristin, would you mind explaining to Bob what we talked about?" Better to let the professional deliver the message.

Without hesitation, she started where I had left off. She reminded Bob that he had not been happy at Mind Boosters and then checked with him to make sure that was the case. He offered no disagreement. She suggested that if he agreed to try the Adult Day program, it would be a big help to me. At the time, I couldn't see how this would be the case, with the additional driving, but if it improved her argument, I was all for it. She finished by asking, "Would you be willing to do that for Cheri? Just try it a day or two a week at Adult Day and see what happens?" That sentence about "doing it for Cheri" stuck with me and I used it at various times in the future to gain his agreement about a change.

He pondered her question for a few minutes, then finally agreed without enthusiasm. He quickly added, "I'm not doing any crafts, though." Kristin had heard his complaints about crafts when she was with Mind Boosters and knew his aversion well.

But at his reasserting it, we all burst into laughter. Kristin assured him he would not have to do any crafts or any activity he didn't want to do. She teased, "Maybe we can even get a badge to put on your shirt that says, 'I don't do crafts.'" Again, Kristin and I laughed with the relief that Bob was willing to give it a try.

The next week I telephoned Adult Day to let them know we wanted to transfer Bob one day a week but continue with Mind Boosters on Friday. Everyone agreed to the plan, but I learned that enrolling Bob in his new program would require several meetings. It involved a great deal of paperwork starting with the admissions coordinator, then a visit with the nurse on staff, and another meeting with the activities staffer to learn what choices there were for him and what he'd like to sign up for. It would be a while before he could start attending the program.

In the first meeting, I received all the information about the Adult Day program including the daily fee. We were accustomed to a fee for Mind Boosters, but this fee was higher, and of course the more days Bob attended, the more it would cost. The amount, I told myself, was less expensive than hiring a caregiver to come and stay with him the afternoons that I was away from home. Furthermore, the benefits to Bob in a stay-at-home arrangement would be nil. I had already learned that a person with dementia needed social interaction. Isolating him at home would be the worst solution to his Mind Booster difficulties. The day program also had a set routine, which I knew was important. I reassured myself that more activities would be available, some of which Bob would enjoy more than Mind Boosters.

Enrolling in the day program would make Bob eligible for the community paratransit, a benefit I did not expect. A bus would pick him up at our home in the morning and then return him in the afternoon. I was pleased to hear that my chauffeur responsibilities might be reduced.

After all of the meetings and administrative requirements were completed, Bob started his new schedule. The staff encouraged me to attend a part of his first day, and Bob welcomed my coming along. When I picked him up, later that afternoon, I asked, "Well, how did it go?"

"It was great," he answered. His body language showed it. He was relaxed, had no criticism of the day, and told me what the lunch was like—they served a salad, which he loved. After a couple of weeks, Bob asked if he could go more than one day a week. We increased his attendance one day at a time over several weeks until he was going to his new program every day but Friday.

He still wanted to attend Mind Boosters, despite his difficulties with the activities. He continued with both programs for a few weeks until one day after Mind Boosters, in the car on the way home, Bob said, "I don't really want to go to Mind Boosters anymore, but I don't want to just not show up." I knew that when a participant died, that's how everyone knew; they didn't see the person any longer. For whatever reason, the facilitator did not tell the group about a participant's death. I usually found out about a death from someone in my support group or I read it in the local newspaper. I could understand that Bob wouldn't want his friends at Mind Boosters to think he had died.

His timing for leaving Mind Boosters, luckily, happened to be perfect. It was early December, and I knew that Mind Boosters always had a holiday party and invited caregivers to attend. I called the facilitator and told her that Bob had decided to stop attending, but he wanted to return for the annual party. I also said he might want to read some kind of "goodbye" note to his fellow Mind Boosters. She agreed that his reading the note might help complete his transition to the day program.

That evening I told Bob the plan: He would stop attending Mind Boosters but return for the holiday party to say his farewell. I suggested we write something together that he would read to acknowledge his favorite people he had met there and at the same time let others know he would not be attending anymore.

"That sounds great," he said. "When can we write it?"

That night we started a draft and finished it the next day. He knew the people he wanted to recognize but had difficulty forming sentences about their uniqueness. I wasn't surprised. It had been some time since he had written letters or notes, a skill he once prized. For this occasion, we worked well together as we had in previous years — something I had missed. He was open to my suggestions and seemed to enjoy putting his farewell speech together with my guidance.

When the day of the holiday party arrived, Bob wanted to practice reading his farewell before we went. I began to see how this letter was the closure he needed as one of the "charter members" of the group, a title he bestowed on himself with great pride.

Upon arrival, I reminded the facilitator that Bob had something he wanted to say to the group. She remembered and then suggested we join the circle of about 20 people — participants and their caregivers sitting in chairs. She joined the circle too and asked everyone to introduce themselves. I gave Bob a nudge to alert him to the fact that this would be his chance to read his farewell.

When our turn came, I stood and introduced myself first, "I'm Cheri Bailly-Jacobs, and I am Bob's wife and his caregiver." I signaled for him to stand and, after waiting a few minutes to clear his throat, he began to read his farewell. I looked at him with enormous pride, feeling he was so brave to give a speech five years after his diagnosis. Here is Bob's farewell speech.

Merry Christmas & Happy Holidays to Everyone
I'm very glad to be here today. It's been a while since I've seen some of you. I'm now in another program.

But as many of you know, I was a Charter Member

of Mind Boosters. So, today, at the annual party, I'd like to honor just a couple of the members who are no longer with us.

First, Gene who used to always say to me; "You are a card, and you need to be dealt with." I loved Gene.

Next, I remember Les. He always reminded us that he was from Minnesota. We all knew he was a great architect.

I used to love to talk to Ida about New York. As a native New Yorker, she knew all about the places I'd visited.

We all loved Joan, but when I found out her dad was born in my hometown of Davenport, Iowa, that was really great.

Charlie was a WWII hero. I'll never forget when he told us that he survived when his ship went down in the English Channel.

So, it was great to see you all today. Again, Happy Holidays!

After he finished, people applauded. Bob looked so pleased and also ready to leave his treasured Mind Boosters. Another transition was behind us. As I congratulated him, I had to remind myself that there was more to come.

Part Five

Transportation Challenges

CHAPTER 26

The Driving Decision

One of the many unexpected facts we learned about Alzheimer's disease was that the diagnosing physician is required by law in California to report a diagnosis of Alzheimer's to the Department of Motor Vehicles (DMV). It would have sounded the death knell to Bob's ability to drive. Since he was diagnosed as having Mild Cognitive Impairment, there was nothing for us to worry about—for the time being. Since Bob loved to drive, he continued to do so in a limited way.

He drove himself around town to run errands, go to meetings for his volunteer work and Senior Choir rehearsals. From time to time, he did ask me to draw him a map to a location, such as a retirement facility where the choir was going to perform. I gladly drew the map but was concerned that, while he had never gotten lost, my drawings were rudimentary and not a substitute for a navigator in the passenger seat—the role I had played for years. The problem I focused on was helping him get organized enough in advance of an outing so he could drive to a new destination on time. He had developed a habit of arriving late more than usual, and I had explained it to myself as a result of poor planning, not a driving skill deficit.

However, shortly after we started telling friends that Bob was having memory problems, the question, "Is he still driving?" raised its not so pretty head. Whether friends who asked the question were more concerned about Bob's safety or their own was another matter. When I responded (Bob never said a word if he was present), I felt the defensiveness in my chest as I explained, "Yes, but he usually only drives in town. He admits to me that he's afraid to drive on a freeway anymore."

Their questions eventually forced me to ask myself when might he be a danger, not only to himself but to others. Either way, I began to monitor his driving to see if he was making mistakes or taking chances he hadn't before. He usually did all right, unless I interrupted his concentration with a request to make an unplanned turn or stop. I saw that he could not quickly process such interruptions and promised myself to be silent when he was driving.

As the months from the diagnosis turned to years, Bob began to take himself out of the driver's seat. Before we got into the car in the garage, more frequently he would say, "I don't feel like driving today. Do you mind driving?"

Upon reflection sometime later, I had to face the fact that his not wanting to drive on any given day was more than a matter of being tired or short on energy. It was a sign of decline. My old friend "denial" was having its way with me again. If I could tell myself Bob was "just not having a good day," I wouldn't have to face the consequences of his no longer driving at all. Who wants to imagine taking the keys away and saying your driving days are over? Bob would know instantly he had lost his independence and the freedom he so enjoyed.

Finally, one day before I drove out of the driveway with Bob already in the passenger seat, I asked, "Can you describe how you feel when you tell me you don't want to drive?"

He thought for a minute or two and then said, "I just feel kind of fuzzy."

I took that to mean he somehow knew he couldn't think clearly and was even aware he couldn't drive safely. After that brief explanation, I more frequently began to get in on the driver's side of the car, usually checking with him as I started the engine, "Are you okay with me driving?" I didn't want him to think I had taken over without his agreement. Already in the passenger seat, he always nodded a yes. No further discussion was necessary. In time, I became accustomed to being the family driver. This signaled not only a loss of independence for him but a simultaneous loss of freedom for me. I never realized how much I looked forward to going places by myself and enjoying the time alone until I didn't have that freedom any longer. Before, I would plan a trip to go shopping, make my list, and shout down the hallway to Bob, "I'm off. I'll be back in an hour or so. Bye." Now I would walk to him and say, "I'm going to run some errands. Do you want to come with me?" He always did.

I couldn't admit to anyone, even myself, how disappointed his answer made me feel. First, the guilt hit me. He can't go by himself, I scolded myself, so of course he wants to go! The least you can do is to provide an unplanned outing for him. Slowly, I became aware that my disappointment stemmed from two facts: I was not going to get any time alone, and I wouldn't have a break from caregiving.

Running an errand with Bob along meant I would be caregiving as we made our way in and out of the car, in and out of the store, finding a restroom for him, and meeting other needs he might have.

In the late fall of 2005, a standard DMV letter arrived to remind Bob to go through the license renewal process since his license would expire on his birthday, December 16th. Since our agreement had been "no secrets" from the beginning, I knew I had to show it to him but tried to soften the news by saying, "You know you're really not driving anymore, so it will be easy just to let it expire, right?" He had no immediate reaction. Because it was taking him longer and longer to process information, in a sense this was no surprise. I knew the subject was important to him.

Instead of hearing a decision from him, I put the notice in my bill-paying file and tried not to think about it. I told myself Bob wasn't worried, another agreement with myself to keep bad news at bay. Then a week before his birthday, I casually reminded him we weren't renewing his license and sought tacit agreement that this was the plan. Wrong.

"I think I should renew the license, and I'm sure I can pass the test," he confidently announced later that day. My heart sank. I'd been telling everyone who asked about his driving that he wasn't driving anymore. Other caregivers in my support group were struggling with the same issue and were getting more resistance than I was. I had felt lucky Bob had been so compliant.

After a few moments of reflection, I tried the logic approach. "Well, sweetie, you're not driving, so it doesn't make sense to renew your license."

"I'd like to keep it. It's not a problem."

His unusual firmness was not entirely a shock. As I had learned, dementia at this stage can sometimes make people behave much the way they used to. In Bob's case, this meant frank and steadfast about a position; other days, he would lose track of a point in the conversation and walk away. This day Bob was holding firm. I had to do something beyond the fruitlessness of an argument.

Then I had an idea. I reminded him there was a sample test in the back of the driver's manual. I said, "Why don't you take the sample test and see how you do?"

"Okay, that's a great idea," he said as he started for his desk to find the manual.

It wasn't long before he came back into the kitchen, head down, looking unhappy. "How did it go?" I asked cautiously.

"I couldn't answer the questions," he replied with a hangdog look. He was disappointed and probably shocked. He had been a good test taker in college, and he was still doing well with paper and pencil tests at the Alzheimer's Disease Center when he went back for retesting.

Conflicted feelings silenced me. I wanted to comfort him but was relieved to have the driving matter finally resolved: no license, no driving, no accidents. I put my arms around him and asked if he'd like lunch.

It took me a while to comprehend that Bob's giving up on driving had been complicated and different for each of us. I knew how much Bob had enjoyed driving, but I had focused on the practical consequences and inconveniences of being the family driver. I hadn't recognized the loss we both had to accept: Part of the joy in our life together was over. I still think of us on our honeymoon in Italy, him driving our rented VW along the Autostrada, me with my nose buried in the Michelin map telling him what exit to take. We were a great team in the car. Now I was going solo.

By necessity, I came to see this forced independence as growth for me. Doing all the driving put me in control, a feeling I had little of in those days. Yes, more of my freedom and my time alone in the car had disappeared. And yes, almost every loss of Bob's was a loss for me. A loss is painful no matter what. To ignore that feeling was denial—something I was trying to learn to replace with acceptance sooner rather than later.

CHAPTER 27

Who Will Be the Navigator?

I love maps. I didn't discover this about myself until I started to travel with Bob in his healthy days. At the beginning of a road trip, he would place himself behind the steering wheel, having silently appointed himself the sole driver. I would seat myself on the passenger side and search for the appropriate map(s) in the door pocket. If I weren't going to drive, the maps would give me something important to do. And I found I liked being able to answer his questions: "Is the next exit the one we want?" or "Can you tell when this freeway ends?" and of course, "How many miles is it to the next roadside rest area?"

When I began to drive more and more, I assumed Bob would become the designated navigator as I took on the driving. We never discussed this change of roles. I thought he loved maps as much as I did and the new navigator job might be fun for him.

Then we took a trip to Princeton, New Jersey, to visit Bob's son and his family. Since his son picked us up at the airport, driving and navigating were not yet an issue.

We knew from prior visits that as Bob's grandchildren grew and became more active, their noise and ruckus were causing him confusion and anxiety. So, before leaving home, we planned that a break in the middle of the visit would be a good idea. We talked about how I would be doing the driving, especially on the interstate highways. For the site of our break, we chose the Chesapeake Bay region, an area neither of us had visited. Just the idea of learning the area's history made us excited to head out on our own, memory loss and all.

A couple of days into our visit, Bob's son took us to the nearby rental agency to pick up our reserved car. He also gave us clear directions on how to get to the New Jersey Turnpike and the major highway changes we would see leading south to Maryland's Eastern Shore. I glanced at the maps and felt the route would be easy enough. I had never driven on East Coast freeways, though; the narrow width of the roads and speed of the traffic were a bit daunting. I drove cautiously as Bob settled into being a passenger and enjoying the sights from industrial zones to green stretches, with city skylines off in the distance. It sometimes surprised me he didn't ask to drive but said many times what a good driver I was. In our early years together, if I were at the wheel, he would have been pushing to stop and change drivers within a half hour.

By late afternoon, we reached our destination: Easton, Maryland. It was small and quaint with little traffic. With a few missteps, I found our hotel, The Tidewater Inn, a delightful old stand-alone brick building with a small circular driveway and a large dining room for sit-down breakfasts. Bob loved it. I think it reminded him of the travels he had taken with his parents in the 1940s when this kind of hotel was the norm for family travel.

We spent three days exploring the area and eating as much fresh seafood as we could manage. Each morning, I looked at the maps, and together we laid out our day: where to go, where our meals would be, and when we wanted to return to the hotel. Since the weather was hot and humid, we planned our day for frequent breaks, enjoying the uniqueness of each small town. A highlight was the day we spent in Salisbury exploring The Ward Museum of Wildfowl. We both loved birds and had never been to such a museum.

I could see the sadness in Bob's face the morning we were to return to Princeton. He had always had a hard time at the end of a trip. At this stage of the disease, he still loved the newness and anticipation of travel, but the ending was even more difficult than before. I tried to reassure him that we would have a beautiful drive back to Princeton with lunch somewhere along the way. However, even when we were back on the road, I could sense his depression. Before we left Easton, I had looked at the maps, pointed out what highway changes he needed to watch for and alert me to. He nodded he understood, and I was confident I had the changes in my mind, not wanting to be too dependent on him for directions.

However, an hour later, the environs began to look different than what I remembered from our travel south a few days before. Finally, I knew something was wrong when the names on the road signs were not familiar. I asked Bob, "How far are we from that freeway we need to take to the Chesapeake Bay Bridge?" He had the map open on his lap and was staring at it but didn't answer my question. I tried to wait patiently for him to find our location, but as the miles continued to stream by, I began to feel panicky. "Bob, do you know where we are?" I blurted out—more silence.

Finally, he quietly answered, "No."

I lost my temper and swore at him without thinking. I was so panicked that we were irretrievably lost; I quickly started changing lanes and moving to the right to exit. We had told Bob's son we would be back before dark, and I wanted to keep that commitment. I took the next exit and ended up in a suburban area where I temporarily parked on a side street to examine the map. I had no idea where we were, even after I grabbed the map from Bob and tried to make some sense of the town names and highway numbers.

I didn't know it at the time, but my anger stemmed from feeling totally out of control—a sensation I had been keeping at bay when Bob's inabilities caused me frustration or extra time. He sat quietly while I talked out loud to myself to try to locate a route back to the bridge. I took a deep breath and reminded myself there was no critical reason to hurry. Only then did I begin to figure out where we were. The problem was not nearly as big as I had feared. We didn't need to backtrack after all. Quickly back on a freeway, I was relieved to see the bridge signs and knew we would be okay. When we reached the bridge, I was able to apologize for losing my temper and yelling at Bob. But his silence continued the rest of the trip. I think the shame he felt robbed him of any ability to empathize with me or even attempt to offer an apology about his navigation mistake.

During the rest of the drive, I began to reminisce about all the years I had been Bob's co-pilot, but now he couldn't be that for me. I felt a sadness creep over me knowing those wonderful days were gone. I felt alone.

Everyone talks about the loss that a person with dementia experiences, but I was still trying to learn that no one explains how those losses directly affect the partner's life. Yes, people speak of seeing their loved one fade away. Losing the pieces of what made our lives together a partnership hit me in a thousand unexpected ways, including that learning to live with the myriad of changes was a challenge I would face alone.

As the years went by, my confidence in being the responsible party for everything eventually began to grow, and I realized I could take care of most everything on my own and take good care of Bob too.

When I look back on the Chesapeake trip, I mostly recall his earlier advice to me when I would complain about being laid off or inheriting a new boss not of my choosing. He would say, "It's character building, sweetheart."

He was so right. With his disease, I had been granted countless opportunities to build character.

CHAPTER 28

Trials with the Paratransit Bus

The advantages of Bob attending Adult Day were numerous, especially considering the number of additional professionals available to us: registered nurse, occupational therapist, and physical therapist all on site every day. There was a stationary bike in a separate room where he could ride every day. Lastly, the best news for me, the paratransit bus (Vine Go) would transport him to and from Adult Day. I would be free from 9:30 to 3:00 Monday through Friday. The services seemed heaven-sent.

The administrative staff at Adult Day referred me to the paratransit bus service but explained it was up to me to make the arrangements. It sounded simple, but like so many things in those days, it wasn't. I learned that an Adult Day participant qualifies for the bus service only if he is unable to take public transportation (Bob's memory difficulties met this disability requirement) and if the home address is in the paratransit service territory. After I made several phone calls and submitted all the paperwork, I learned we were not in the Vine Go service territory after all, so Bob would not be eligible for the paratransit bus. I, therefore, continued to drive Bob to and from Adult Day.

When friends frequently asked why Bob wasn't taking the bus, I explained we were out of their service area. However, those same friends said they had seen the bus in our neighborhood. Finally, tired of their prodding, I spoke with Adult Day staff about our situation. A staff member, who was knowledgeable about every aspect of the program, volunteered to contact the bus service herself and straighten everything out. She too was confident the bus should be able to provide transport for Bob. We never knew what the problem had been, but she resolved it.

On the last Friday in March of 2009, we were told Vine Go would pick up Bob the following Monday. There was no charge for the service, but by now, I had lost some confidence in Napa's public transportation bureaucracy.

With some apprehension, because any change in Bob's routine gave him anxiety, I told him that Monday would be his first bus day. He seemed pleased at first, but then he asked me several times during the weekend when would the bus come. I was now accustomed to this repetitive and slightly anxious questioning, and I had learned not to tell him anything too far in advance, as that would create more anxiety. Even telling him on that Friday turned out to be too soon.

The document I received when Bob was approved for the bus listed an additional rule for participants: The passenger had to be ready for pickup 15 minutes before the scheduled arrival time. Although the schedule was set, since each passenger had different needs, the arrival time could vary depending on which riders used the service. Being ready in advance made sense.

That Monday, more than 15 minutes before pick-up time, Bob was dressed, fed, and excited for his first bus ride. We stood at the end of the driveway and waited. And waited. Bob finally said, "I don't like waiting for a bus." He must have been remembering his days as a kid in Davenport, Iowa, when he took the bus downtown by himself. This day the bus never came.

Trying to be upbeat, I smiled at him as we went back in the house, but I feared this might be the beginning of his unwillingness to use the bus even if it were to come. In some distress, I telephoned the Adult Day office. There had been a miscommunication. It turned out Vine Go only made bus schedule changes the first of the month, so Bob would not be on the schedule for another two days, since this Monday was March 30. Working hard not to show him my frustration with what I determined to be bureaucratic regulations, I returned to my chauffeur role, driving Bob once more to the other end of town for his Adult Day activities.

On Wednesday, April 1, the bus arrived early for Bob's first trip. Instead of the relief I thought I would feel, apprehension crept into my chest. It had been a long time since Bob went anywhere without me. We walked up the driveway to meet the driver, who had already gotten out of the bus.

"Hi, Bob. I've been waiting to meet you."

His friendliness immediately reassured me. Bob was not just a name on a list to him. I introduced myself and asked him his name. He said he was Sean and we shook hands. He turned his attention to Bob again, welcoming him and helping him board. He said, as he put him in the front seat, he wanted Bob to have the best view, then mouthed quietly to me he could keep an eye on him there.

As he assisted Bob, I explained that Bob took a salad with him every day but was unable to keep track of his lunch box. Still holding the lunch box, I asked, "What is the best thing to do?" Sean said he would keep it up front and give it directly to one of the staff members when they arrived at Adult Day. It seemed like a simple request, but hard to ask for like so many other times. Relieved, I handed him the box. Bob would have forgotten it, and that would have caused other problems.

Meanwhile, I recognized the fellow across the aisle from Bob as a quiet, younger participant who used to open the front door for me at Adult Day each time I went to pick up Bob. I smiled at him and said, "Hi." He raised one hand but said nothing. I was glad I'd been friendly to him before, for he looked like the kind of guy no one wanted to look in the eye. I liked that I could have a genuine smile on my face, although he never smiled back. This soundless exchange became our routine every morning. It was something I would have shared with Bob in our early days, but now I knew he wouldn't be able to understand the significance of such a simple connection for me.

That first day, another man sitting behind Bob told me not to forget to pick up the newspaper in our driveway. It was the least essential task for me on this important morning, but I was growing used to small matters being foremost in these troubled brains. I simply said, "Thank you."

As the bus pulled away, Sean waved while Bob looked straight ahead. I knew I was out of his awareness, that his attention was focused on the road and the ride. Telling myself he was safe, I picked up the newspaper and started to walk back to the house. As soon as I opened the door to the kitchen, I started to cry — part relief, part sadness. It was like putting a child on the train to visit grandparents for the first time. I was glad Bob was open to this new adventure, but I wasn't ready to trust him on his own and felt a melancholy I didn't understand. The extra hours in the morning and afternoon I didn't have to drive Bob to and from Adult Day were a welcome reprieve. So where was my expected wave of "free again"?

The bus routine soon became a significant part of our morning preparation. Every morning, Bob was ready on time and made his way to my office to wait. He stared out of the French doors for the bus like a child waiting for the rain to stop. If the bus was late, he grew anxious and suggested I call and check on it. Instead, I would sit with him, usually just a few minutes. "There's the bus coming around the corner, Bob." With that news, he was up on his feet and heading for the front door.

Lucky for us, Sean was the regular driver in the morning and often walked to meet us halfway down the driveway. One day, I saw him massaging his shoulder as if he were experiencing some pain. When he saw Bob, though, he smiled and said, "Hi, Bob. I feel better every morning when I see you." He helped him up the stairs and into the seat while continuing to talk to me. "I wish all my passengers were as nice as Bob. If they were, this would be a great job. He is always a gentleman." I noticed Sean had stopped rubbing his shoulder.

Bob didn't react to these comments. I think his attention was focused on the bus stairs. But as I waved goodbye, I thought how great it was that Bob, a person with so few abilities now, could still bring joy to another human by just being a gentleman and giving a genuine smile. I was unusually proud of him that day.

After he had been riding the bus for months, without explanation, he asked me for a card to take with him. I wasn't quite sure what his concern was. I ventured a guess. "Do you want something written down so if someone needs to know who you are or where you are going, they could read the card?"

"Yes," he said. "That would be good."

It was another surprise for me. I had no idea he was worried about being lost on the bus trip. I picked up one of the 3 x 5 cards on the kitchen island that I regularly used to write out his daily schedule. He watched me as I carefully printed: My name is Bob Jacobs. I take the Vine Go bus to Adult Day Health Program on South Jefferson Street in the morning. In the afternoon I take the bus to my home at Revere Circle in Napa.

"Is this what you were wanting?" I asked as I handed him the card.

"That's perfect, " he said with a smile as he put the card in his shirt pocket.

In those latter days of Bob's disease, caregiving was especially difficult. I was grateful to be able to help reduce his worry and anxiety in whatever way I could, although he didn't usually offer any recognition for the help I gave him. I had learned that he needed his full concentration to accomplish the smallest tasks. The hard lesson for me was that his awareness of me or what I did was beyond him. His smile on this occasion seemed to reflect appreciation, which sustained me for another day of caregiving.

CHAPTER 29

Unexpected Lessons from an Auto Accident

There were times when I still needed to drive Bob to or from Adult Day, even with the bus service. And we didn't have any arrangements with other participants to share the transportation as we did at Mind Boosters.

After dropping him off and before picking him up, I developed the bad habit of using these car trips as a brain break—driving almost mindlessly—70% present in the vehicle and 30% somewhere else in time and space. My excuse for this distracted driving was that by early October of 2007, I was five years into being a caregiver, which meant I was usually tired and full of feelings I didn't want to have. I was easily angered, feeling both our lives were too often out of control, and lonely for the Bob I knew and loved.

One autumn afternoon, as I exited the freeway and turned onto Imola Avenue, a wide boulevard with numerous freeway exits and entrances, I checked my watch to make sure I was on time to pick up Bob. Then three blocks ahead, I saw a pickup truck stopped in my lane for no apparent reason. I came back to reality just in time to brake and avoid causing an accident. Luck was on my side, I thought. However, as I glanced in my rearview mirror, I saw a small red sports car barreling down on me. Having stopped right behind the pickup left me no room to turn into the adjacent lane and avoid the oncoming car. My hands froze on the steering wheel, and I held my head hard against the headrest just in time for the sports car to slam into my car's rear end.

Stunned, I sat there for a minute. My first thought was how could I get my car out of the middle of the street. My second thought was I'm going to be late to pick up Bob. What do I do now? The sports car backed up after colliding with me, and I managed to drive across the street and park near the corner. Before I could get out of my car, a tall young man jumped out of the sports car and ran toward me. He shouted, "I'm sorry. I'm so sorry. Are you all right?" I must have been experiencing mild shock as I wasn't even angry that my Honda had been rear-ended.

Minutes later, to my further confusion, the young man's mother arrived on the scene in another car. I soon learned she was the owner of the sports car, and her son must have called her on his cell phone immediately after the accident.

She was out of her car in a flash and also started apologizing about the accident and asking if I was okay. She quickly introduced herself and added that she was a nurse at the local hospital. That explained her persistence in asking about my condition. I blurted out I thought I was all right and managed to say, "My husband is at a facility a few blocks away, and he's expecting me to pick him up." At the same time, I realized I had left my cell phone at home, and I didn't have the number of the Adult Day office. I felt ashamed for being so unprepared. And I couldn't think clearly. Only much later did I realize I was probably suffering from mild shock.

Another man who had witnessed the accident stopped his car and came up to me to offer help. I asked him to call Adult Day. He readily agreed, but since I didn't have their number he was unable to contact them. (In my confusion/shock I couldn't recall the formal name of Adult Day for anyone to search for the number.)

The mother offered to drive me to pick up Bob and drive me back to the scene of the accident, where I could exchange insurance information with her son. I had a rush of feelings about leaving my car. I couldn't seem to think straight. Since only the rear end was damaged, I wasn't worried about being able to drive it if I could figure out what to do about Bob. A city police officer had appeared on the scene but didn't seem to take charge.

I was also concerned about getting into a car with a total stranger while still trying to figure out the best thing to do next. I felt embarrassed that I had never made a plan for Bob's transportation in case I had an accident or car trouble. And why wasn't I carrying my phone? The self-criticism arrived along with the adrenaline. Reluctantly, I accepted the mother's offer.

When we arrived at Adult Day a few minutes later, I asked the stranger/mother/nurse to wait in the car, explaining I would locate Bob and alert Adult Day about the accident. If Bob started to worry about why I hadn't come to pick him up, he might become anxious and create even more difficulties for me when I did arrive.

I hurried into the building and looked for one of the social workers. Out of the corner of my eye, I saw Bob sitting in his usual place in the lobby looking calm and content. He was with others waiting to be picked up. I was confident he hadn't seen me arrive. I saw Sheila, the social worker, standing nearby and headed in her direction.

"Sheila, can you help me?" I asked. She led me toward a more private place where we could talk. In the past, she had advised us about so many situations, seeing her helped me realize she would be the perfect person to ask for assistance.

She quickly responded, "Of course, Cheri. Are you okay?" I must have looked frazzled even though I was trying to keep myself together.

"Yes, but I had a car accident down on Imola, just blocks from here. I don't want to take Bob there, and I don't want him wondering where I am. I can drive the car, but I didn't want to be late picking him up. What should I do?" I asked. The tears I had been holding back surfaced and streamed down my cheeks.

She glanced over at Bob and then turned to me, "I'll move Bob to another location so he won't keep looking for you to come through the front door. I'll tell him you're running late and you called to alert us that you'll be here soon." I felt immediate relief that she knew how to manage the situation and not cause him anxiety or fear.

"Thank you so much, Sheila. I'm going to go get the car, and I'll be back soon," I managed to tell her. I walked quickly to the mother's car in the parking lot, and minutes later we were back at the accident scene.

We exchanged all the necessary information. Mother and son both seemed relieved I was not hurt nor angry. They had no idea that my brain was wired to worry about Bob, not myself, and certainly not the car. I was confident their insurance would be responsible for repairing it. We finished the information exchange in less than 30 minutes.

When I returned to pick up Bob, he was his usual cheerful self at seeing me. He had no idea about the accident, and we drove home as if nothing had happened.

When I had time to regroup, I told him about the accident, minimizing emotions as best I could. I missed being able to vent to him and receive his support. The abbreviated story of the crash didn't seem to faze him. That was the positive side of Alzheimer's—things that did not involve Bob directly didn't usually have an observable effect.

For me, however, that evening I experienced a different kind of understanding. As I retraced the day's events, I had to accept a new reality; I could not always be in control. My therapist was right. I could ask for help even though I had long thought I was the one good in an emergency. I used to tell people I had a migraine personality: I could get everyone through a crisis and afterward have a blistering migraine. Today, however, I had told someone I respected, Sheila, that I didn't know what to do and needed her to step in and think for me. And she did.

My therapist was right—I *could* ask for help. She had said making yourself vulnerable by asking for help is something you need to learn to do if you are to continue to care for Bob and experience the growth that is possible for you. Today was a chance for me to try out her teaching.

Part Six

A Break Rather Than a Breaking Point

CHAPTER 30

My Fears about Alzheimer's Camp

ob brought home a flyer from Adult Day that announced a respite weekend would take place in late April at Enchanted Hills, a camp on Mount Veeder above the Napa Valley. In the world of chronic illnesses, the word respite usually meant relief for caregivers from the responsibilities of caregiving for a few hours or a few days. As I read on, I happily learned the camp was for people with memory problems, and indeed the blessed respite was for caregivers like me.

The notice included instructions about dates and times for the participants and their drivers. Campers were to arrive Friday after 3:00 and be picked up early afternoon on Sunday. For me, this meant a free weekend, a break from all responsibilities for caregiving. My anticipated gratitude and excitement were a challenge to keep in check.

Before I called the number for more information, I knew I needed to talk with Bob first. That afternoon in our living room, while he was sitting at his desk, I casually asked, "Would you be interested in going to a camp for the weekend? The flyer says it's for people with memory loss." I held my breath as I waited for him to respond. I was reasonably confident he had not read it before giving it to me.

Finally, he said, "Sure."

I was amazed. Part of my caution came from knowing that before his memory and cognitive decline, Bob's idea of going to the woods might mean a stay at a lovely inn or a historic lodge in a state park, but not a camp. And he had told me years earlier that his mother had never permitted him to go to summer camp as a kid. He seemed to have no questions and continued to busy himself with whatever was on his desk. The conversation seemed so inconsequential to him that I may as well have asked, "Do you want chicken for dinner?"

I said, "Okay, I'll get more details." I didn't want to create any doubts where there seemed to be none. His customary trust encouraged me to continue finding such resources. Now, Bob had hand-delivered one to me.

I called Adult Day and signed up Bob for the camp. To my surprise, there were no fees; donations to the agency paid for everything, and volunteers assisted the campers.

When the promised packet of information arrived in the mail, it was full of detailed instructions: "Label all clothing items, label all personal items (shaver, brush, toothpaste, etc.), and put all prescription drugs in their original containers." Since I didn't know if any medical professionals would be at the camp, I was concerned about Bob's medications. He was accustomed to having his pills in his weekly organizer and my giving them to him at the appropriate time.

I was annoyed that the instructions meant more tasks for me to do. Wasn't I the one in need of a break? Now I faced an additional project to finish before getting that break.

My concern about his medications was for naught; I learned later that a nurse would administer them. This made sense, but of course the Sunday through Saturday pill container I had already filled would be useless. My annoyance, partnered with impatience, grew. The early spring weather did not help.

As the departure weekend drew near, it began to rain every day, all day. Bob didn't say anything about it. Neither did I. Although it was a short 45-minute drive from the valley floor up to the camp, I knew the road — narrow and full of curves — would be compromised from all the rain. Leaving Bob in the care of other people overnight in a different and unfamiliar environment was a new experience for me. I spent a lot of mental time reassuring myself that I was doing the right thing for him and me.

Finally, the first day of the camp arrived. It rained so hard all morning; I felt I had to check with Bob to see if he still wanted to go. "Of course," he answered, as if there were no reason not to go. I wasn't sure if he was aware it was rainy and cold, but I felt I had done the right thing to check with him. I felt some guilt about not pointing out to him how stormy the weather conditions were. Not enough, though, to give him my usual verbose explanation of why I was asking.

In the years before he became ill, the weather was a topic we would have had many conversations about: Would the skies clear? What clothes should we take to keep ourselves warm? The silence in our lives now made it hard for me to know if I was doing the right thing for either or both of us. Until this coming weekend, I didn't realize how dependent

I had become on all the words that once connected us in our daily lives.

Early Friday afternoon, we began to pack the car. It was easy, unlike previous car trips, as there was nothing for me to pack for myself. After lunch, I asked Bob if he was ready to go, and his enthusiasm for the weekend was evident as he headed for the garage with no need for a reminder or encouragement from me.

As we started up into the hills of the west side of the valley (where the rain can be torrential) the skies grew darker. The rain was incessant and had taken its toll. My worst fears about road conditions were confirmed: edges of the road had washed away, holes in the roadbed were everywhere, and rocks had slid down the hills onto the roadway.

I looked at Bob to see if he was upset by the road conditions, but he seemed calm, looking out the window as if we were on a Sunday drive on a sunny spring day. The difference in our attitudes toward the trip was similar to many of our days now; I was anxious and concerned about everything, and he was living in a child's world where everything was taken care of by a loving parent.

I glanced in the mirror and saw a look on my face that said, "What are we doing?" I struggled the whole trip with my decision to take Bob into the wilderness, as I thought of it, in such terrible weather. A couple of times I said to him, "How are you doing, babe?"

He calmly responded, "Fine," and I believed him.

Finally, I saw the sign for Enchanted Hills and turned down a steep, narrow private road that led to a flat area with surrounding buildings and a small pond. As I stole a look at Bob, there were still no signs of fear on his face. It reminded me of how much travel had meant to him in our years together. Even now, when he didn't know where we were going, the trip was a welcome adventure.

After I found the parking area, I felt the relief of our safe arrival, but a lump in my throat emerged and the reproach in my heart reappeared. Had I arranged this weekend for selfish reasons? Was I leaving Bob with people I might not even know so that I could have some time without him? Mostly, yes.

We moved his things out of the car. He was busy looking around, and he never saw the couple in the car next to us. I didn't know them, but by now I recognized the vacant look on the face of the man who had some form of dementia. Bob, however, did not seem aware of anything except the meadow below us and cabins nearby. I was so grateful he had stayed positive, given the rain and the drive. I didn't think to give myself any credit for arranging the weekend. I was concerned about what might happen next when he saw the facilities and accommodations, not the five-star resort he may have been expecting.

We made our way to the drab and rustic one-story dormitory. A team from Adult Day and Mind Boosters greeted us. I recognized a couple of the staff and appreciated their friendly, open response to him. "Hi, Bob. You made it. Welcome to camp!"

They led us into the dorm and showed us his assigned room. My apprehension grew as I realized I thought Bob would have his own bedroom. Instead, the sleeping space had three cots and was surprisingly monastic. His roommates were already there and welcomed him, though none of them knew each other.

I kept an eye on him as I unpacked his things, found a temporary home for most of them, and tried to explain to

Bob where I had put them. He either couldn't concentrate on details or was too excited to be at the camp; so again, I was the only one who had concerns.

One of the supervisors came to show him the location of the showers, lavatories, and the community room. It seemed like this was a signal for me to depart. Before he left on the tour, I quickly hugged him, but I could tell his mind was on the tour. He seemed so upbeat. I reassured him I would be back to pick him up on Sunday and told him, "Have fun." He barely noticed I was leaving.

Once I reached the car, I began to relax. I felt like I had been holding my breath since we left home. With that breathing came the tears I had also been holding back. I sat in the car and cried quietly without caring if someone might see me. Eventually, I felt calm enough to drive. I started the car and headed up the steep hill out of the camp, afraid to look back for fear the tears would reappear, and I didn't want to stop halfway up the hill on the single-lane road.

The return trip to the valley floor seemed faster than the recent ascent. I was off on my free weekend. Once back in town, I stopped at the store to get fun food for snacks and to rent the latest videos for my weekend entertainment.

Back home, I immediately noticed how different it was not to have Bob in the house. At first, the rooms felt bare and hollow. I realized I had grown accustomed to listening for him, wondering what was he doing, expecting him to pop into the kitchen any minute. It took a few hours to disconnect the caregiver radar I had developed.

I had no plan for the weekend. I didn't have to do anything or go anywhere, and I didn't. First, I took a nap, a long one. Preparing dinner for myself was a solitary experience after all the years of sharing the kitchen with Bob. I spent

Saturday reading a good book and watching a movie that evening. About the time I became used to the quiet in the house, the weekend was over, as was the rain. I drove back to Enchanted Hills early Sunday afternoon, enjoying the silence in the car and the sunshine that had thankfully reappeared.

Once at the camp, I found Bob in the community room singing with the other campers, a big smile on his face. That alone told me he'd had a good time, and I couldn't wait to hear about the whole experience. On our drive home, he let me know he was too tired to talk but reassured me that he had had a great time, and the food was fabulous.

Bob returned to the annual camp for the next three years. Each time it was easier for me to leave him. After that first year, I was more confident he would be all right, and I increasingly and desperately craved time alone to do nothing. The 48-hour break was barely enough to meet that need, but it was a start.

Arranging for that first respite from caregiving was intimidating, so I was all the more grateful for a successful first experience. It helped me recognize how important it was to care not only for Bob but myself.

CHAPTER 31

A Failed Getaway Weekend

I began to yearn for a getaway weekend with Bob in the spring of 2007. Our travel the year before had included a trip to Memphis to see family and a fall visit to Davenport, Iowa, for Bob's 60th high school class reunion, but we hadn't gone to a relaxing vacation spot. Both trips had demanded a lot of energy on my part, and I began to realize how much I needed a break. As I sat at my desk and tried to figure out what was the easiest short trip for us to take, I recalled how important travel had been in our lives.

In 1991, 1992, and 1993, we went to Europe for our annual vacation, usually a three-week journey by car to European countries. We explored England, Germany, Ireland, Scotland, and France—automobile trips organized and arranged by Bob. I loved traveling with him, as his curiosity was endless, and he was always open to whatever the journey presented. However, as Bob's disease progressed, travel became more difficult. I frequently had to figure out how to deal with his physical and cognitive difficulties. Walking through airports, understanding what was going on, unfamiliar restrooms, etc. made any trip hard on both of us.

Bob had begun to suffer bouts of anxiety, especially when the surroundings were unfamiliar to him. He became so nervous he couldn't concentrate on anything, and instead he paced wherever we were. I knew that this trip-to-be might be the last time for us to take a real vacation—not just to visit family. I concluded a car trip might be the best thing now. He had always loved putting everything imaginably useful in the car and driving away as if we might never come back. I frequently asked, "Are you taking that too?"

He would explain that when you took a car trip, you really could take everything because you never knew what you might need. "That is the beauty of it!" he said.

But things had changed. Now I would be doing the packing, all the driving, and there would be many stops as Bob would need a restroom frequently.

I broached Bob about the subject of a car trip. My suggestion for this vacation was Carmel. He only took a few seconds to say he thought it was a great idea. I reassured him it would be familiar territory and would be fun to revisit some of our many haunts. He agreed and seemed pleased to have a trip in the offing.

The day we left on our mini-vacation, Bob was his old self. He was excited to get up and tried to help as best he could with packing the car, wanting to take everything, of course, and couldn't wait until we were on the road.

The drive took a couple of hours. In the passenger seat, Bob was glued to the view out his window. As we drove down the east side of San Francisco Bay, he seemed proud that he could remember so many landmarks: "There's the turnoff to Niles Canyon," and near Gilroy, "I remember playing on the Gavilan golf course." Farther along the freeway, "We used to get gas there, remember?" I was impressed with how well his visual memory was working. I took it as a positive sign for the trip.

After we arrived and checked into our hotel, both of us were tired, so we took a well-deserved nap. In the early evening, we headed to the quaint town of Pacific Grove. Our destination was a small organic food restaurant named Tillie Gort that we had frequented years before. I was looking forward to a good wholesome meal and relaxing over it, knowing the setting would be familiar to Bob.

He seemed at ease as we entered the reception area, but as we waited for our meal to arrive, I began to see signs of his anxiety. He stopped talking and seemed fidgety. He was also irritated by the lowering sun in his eyes from the window facing the street and asked me to change seats with him. I reluctantly got up, after reminding him that such glare caused me to get headaches, but he was insistent. The old Bob would never have asked me to tolerate anything that might cause me a migraine. I realized he had forgotten about my headaches and couldn't help that his agitation had consumed his positive mood.

We made it through dinner without further incident and the next day returned to Pacific Grove for a walk through a beautiful park with ocean views, where we had picnicked many times. Today, however, the wind blew fiercely and seemed to create additional irritation for Bob. I asked a couple of times, "Are you okay?" He said yes but then blurted out that he had to go to the restroom. With none in sight, I reluctantly suggested we give up on the walk and head to the village area for some lunch where there would be a restroom. He agreed. We reversed our direction and braced ourselves against the wind as we returned to the car.

We chose the Victorian Corner for lunch, a familiar café, but Bob's main concern was the restroom. Before we even ordered, he announced he needed to visit the men's room. He was gone so long I began to plan what I was going to do if he didn't come back to the table soon. Then he did return, looking frustrated and upset. "I couldn't find the light in there, so I just had to go anyway."

"Did you find the toilet in the dark?"

"I'm not sure," he confessed.

I had visions of a restroom with urine all over the floor and me finding the manager so I could volunteer to mop it up. He seemed reluctant to give me any details and was losing patience with everything. I interrogated him enough to understand he had not made a mess but was angry about not finding the light switch. By now, I was feeling intolerant and couldn't find a way to reconnect with him. We ate our lunch in an uncomfortable silence.

The next day, we went to another familiar site, Point Lobos State Reserve, for a walk on the coast trail. I asked Bob to use his walker since I couldn't remember how rough the trail was. He grudgingly agreed as I removed the walker from the trunk. It was another windy day but sunny and beautiful. After no more than 15 minutes, we reached a viewpoint and stopped to enjoy the scene of the translucent ocean and powerful waves. Bob said, "I think I've had enough."

I could sense his disappointment at not being able to walk the whole trail and thought a suggestion of lunch might brighten his spirits. I began to feel distressed as I realized how often I was scrambling to make his day better, losing sight of my own need for relaxation.

"How about driving out to Carmel Valley and having lunch there?" He agreed but was withdrawn throughout the drive. I realized he might have felt the walk was another athletic activity he used to do with ease. Now it was gone too.

We found an old café in the center of Carmel Valley and decided to eat on the deck to enjoy the fresh air. During lunch, he continued to be quiet, even though I knew he was enjoying his quiche and salad. I asked, "Do you want to drive around here a bit and see what else we can find from our old days?"

"No," he said, "I want to go back."

I decided not to ask for an explanation. Bob was not in a mood to talk. I paid the bill and we left. Driving in silence back to Carmel, I began to realize I had made a mistake in thinking that familiar scenes with lots of memories would be pleasing to him. Maybe they made him feel a loss instead of joy. Or maybe his anxiety was coming on even stronger. Whatever was affecting his disposition, there was no way for me to distract him from it or help him with it, a situation frustrating for him and me.

As soon as we arrived back at the hotel, Bob headed for the bathroom. After that, all he wanted was to lie down. I had brought his "boom box" from home and put on his favorite Mozart CD, hoping it would soothe him. He did sleep for a while, but his frequent trips to the bathroom interrupted any real rest he might have gotten.

I spent most of the afternoon reading, as well as trying to figure out what to do next. Although he had been withdrawn since we arrived in Carmel, the only way I knew to connect with Bob was to talk with him. It's what I'd done for years.

That evening, I crawled in bed with him and put my arms around him. Sometimes he liked that and sometimes he didn't. It was a chance I was taking. Then I said, "Did it make you sad to go to all those places where we had so much fun in our early days?" He nodded. I saw tears in his eyes. I continued, "Because you don't think we'll ever have those days again?"

He said, "Yeah."

I told him it was a loss for me too, and I started to cry. Then I decided to take one more step. I didn't know if I'd have another chance.

I said, "My therapist told me it would be helpful if we could grieve together for what we've both lost. Would you be willing to talk about that a bit?" He nodded again. After we held each other for a long while in silence, we were able to talk quietly about our first years together. He couldn't add much detail, but I knew he was following me as I recalled some of our early travels.

In a wonderful moment, Bob thanked me for this special time. He was able to express how much he appreciated the insight into loss. I was grateful, as well, for it helped me realize that Carmel weekends were a significant loss for me too—yet another I had not anticipated.

We then decided to cut this getaway shorter than planned. We packed up in the morning and headed home. It was where Bob was most comfortable and where Bob and I still had a life together. I also needed quiet time to think how I could find a way to restore some energy and postpone the burnout I feared was not far away.

CHAPTER 32

We Explore Respite Facilities

I loved the time each year when Bob would go to Enchanted Hills for the camp weekend, and I would have 48 delicious hours of respite. But by 2008, after almost seven years of increasingly demanding caregiving, I had to face facts: I needed an extended break more often than once a year, and responsible planning said I needed a place for Bob if for some reason I couldn't care for him. It was hard to admit that I not only craved extended time alone, but I feared I might be approaching burnout. Such admissions felt like I was admitting premature failure. In many ways, Bob was still healthy, and I was aware my caregiving responsibilities would not end soon.

With feelings of fatigue and weariness I could no longer ignore, I decided to search for a respite facility where Bob could try a short stay. By now, I hoped that just doing nothing and staying home alone might replenish some of my energy. Whatever facility I found could go on a list of considerations for a permanent stay, should the need arise.

I began the project by first talking to Bob and explaining we didn't know what the future would bring. We had no family member in the area who could step in for me in the event I could physically no longer care for him. It was difficult for Bob to grasp the concept of my not being his caregiver. Recently, Bob's son, who lived with his family in London at this time, offered to pay for a respite stay to give me a break. The offer was generous and welcome—one I thought we should take advantage of.

As we talked about finding a facility, I saw that he had not imagined that anything could happen that would change our current arrangement. I became even more convinced I needed to find a location that would be safe, familiar, and that he liked.

Despite his lack of comprehension, he was agreeable. "Yeah, I'd like to look at some places."

I decided to start with the size of the facility. Would he prefer a small facility like a house with just two or three bedrooms (usually referred to as a board and care place) or a large facility where there might be activities and more people (now known as memory care or a dementia care facility)? I was amazed at his ready answer, "I think I'd like the place where there would be activities." The positive influence of his Adult Day group experiences was evident.

I looked up the addresses of places I had heard about that provided dementia care. I chose three facilities in different areas of Napa. I did not want to overwhelm him with too many choices. For our initial search, I suggested a version of our favorite outing: a Sunday drive. It had been a childhood ritual for us both.

On the next Sunday, we drove by each of the possible facilities. They all looked more like small hotels than hospitals, which was a plus. At the last one, I told Bob, "I'd like to go in and see if they'll give us a tour. Do you want to come with me?"

I knew he always wanted to go with me wherever I went, but I wasn't sure if a potential place to live would elicit the same open response.

"Sure. I want to see what it looks like inside too." What a trooper he still was. I had been concerned that at some point in our drive, he might start to imagine having to move away from home, and fear would block his natural inquisitiveness.

In we went. The lobby was large with a couch and two chairs, but it felt empty. We waited a bit, taking in all that we could see in the adjacent common area. Finally, someone approached us and asked if we needed help. When I asked for a tour, we learned that no one was available; we would need to call in advance to set up an appointment. I was disappointed but didn't feel we had wasted our time. We had accomplished one important thing: by noticing the gloomy ambiance of the lobby, I could not imagine suggesting Bob go there even for a respite stay and did not set up an appointment for a tour.

After our drive, I asked other caregivers and staff at Adult Day if they knew of a facility that allowed a short respite stay. No one had ever heard of any nor had anyone researched such possibilities. So I explored the Internet for "dementia care facilities near Napa." The more I read about their offerings, the more I wanted to see the places and ask questions I had about their services and prices.

One facility, about an hour away in an adjoining county, did offer respite care for short stays. I called and made an appointment. Then I talked with Bob and asked if he wanted to go with me to see the place. He did, of course.

When we arrived at the facility, I felt nervous but didn't want it to show for fear that Bob would pick up on my mood. As usual those days, he let me take the lead. After we announced ourselves to the receptionist, she said a manager would be with us shortly. As I looked around the sunny, bright reception area and noticed how clean and new everything looked, my nervousness disappeared. The furniture, walls, and floors were attractive and designed as a nice hotel would be.

In a few minutes, the manager appeared, carrying a large stack of papers. She led us to a conference room, obviously meant for a board of directors' meeting. I had expected a cozy room where Bob would be comfortable and our conversation, of a confidential nature, could take place. It felt more like a business meeting than a visit to find care for a loved one, but Bob did not seem put off. The manager queried him about having a roommate or not and what activities interested him. He chatted easily with her. I was taken aback when he said he would prefer to have a roommate. He later told me he couldn't imagine being alone in an unfamiliar room. As surprised as I was by his answer, I learned I needed to continue to ask his opinion and not assume what he might like or dislike.

After we talked for an hour and asked and answered lots of questions, I felt confident enough to settle on five days for his first stay. Then the manager gave us a tour. The building was divided into two sections: one for assisted-living and one for dementia care. On the dementia side, there was a community room where older people were participating in an activity with a leader. It consisted solely of tossing a ball back and forth in a circle. I found the activity simplistic and knew Bob did more than that at Adult Day.

Later, the manager suggested we stay for lunch to give Bob a chance to try the food. We sat in a small dining room by ourselves; we agreed the food was good but not great. By the end of our meal, I could see that Bob was beginning to fade. I located the manager, finalized what would happen next, and made an appointment for another visit, at which I would fill out all the necessary papers.

Then she alerted us to the fact that Bob would need a medical statement from his doctor confirming the details of his health status. That report had to be completed by the doctor no more than 30 days before his visit began. I swallowed my frustration. Like everything else I tried to do for Bob (and myself) to make the caregiving journey more manageable, it took more work before I would feel any relief. Now I had to get Bob an appointment with the doctor in time to coordinate with the dates we had already committed to for his stay.

Our next meeting a week later resulted in further frustration for me. The manager, toting her same stack of papers, now explained we had to complete them all as if Bob were signing up to be a permanent resident. When I questioned this, she said they didn't have forms specifically for a short stay and that the state required this. From my human resources experiences, I knew companies sometimes told a "white lie" that forms were required by government regulation when it was the company's choice to request such documentation. Bob's comfort or anything related to our needs was not the subject of the paperwork. The forms took an hour and a half to complete. Bob was exhausted, but we were on our way to the first stay in a facility.

We left the building with some feeling of accomplishment. Driving home, I began to think about the lengthy "To

Do" list for his first visit: schedule a doctor's appointment to confirm his health status, gather the extensive number of items to be packed, label all items with his name, communicate with Adult Day about Bob's absence, check all his prescriptions, and order refills if necessary. Lastly, we were encouraged to bring any items "for comfort," as the directions read. He chose his boom box and classical music CDs, as well as the small table lamp from his childhood which he frequently kept on at night.

When departure day arrived, Bob seemed excited as if he were going on a vacation trip. Things seemed to be coming together, except for the tickle in the back of my throat that I noticed upon awakening.

Checking Bob into the facility was easy enough. His mood seemed positive and relaxed. After moving his belongings into his room, however, I began to feel shaky. When it was time to say goodbye, I felt like crying but didn't want to show my tears in front of him because he seemed so positive. Instead, I gave him a quick hug and said, "Have fun. I'll see you in a few days."

With the supervisor standing close by, I was confident Bob was safe, although he now gave me an odd look that said he wasn't quite sure what was happening.

As I walked out the door, tears quietly streamed down my cheeks. I couldn't wait to get to the privacy of the car. There, as with my first time taking Bob to Enchanted Hills, I allowed myself finally to feel the complicated emotions I had been pushing away: guilt for choosing my needs over what he might feel, relief to be free of caregiving responsibilities, and sadness at the reality that he needed 24-hour supervision.

I drove straight home, went to bed, and slept most of the day. My throat was getting worse. I self-diagnosed a cold on the way; the first I had contracted in years. I spent most of the five-day respite in bed. Although I knew that was the best care I could give myself, I was disappointed there was no time for any fun. And I wanted to be well for Bob's return. Furthermore, I missed him. That I received no calls from the facility was a good sign. Still sniffling when I picked him up, he seemed cheery and glad to see me. He didn't notice my cold, and I didn't tell him, not wanting him to worry about catching it.

Of course, as was my habit, I peppered him with questions on the way home. "What did you like best?" I asked.

"The bus rides," he said.

"What bus rides?

"Every day we went on a bus ride around different places in Sonoma County. The driver was such a nice guy," he added.

I had one more question, "Did you make any friends there?"

A long silence followed by "Uh-huh, the bus driver." Not the answer I had expected. If he had been able to make new friends, the next respite might be easier for me to suggest.

When we arrived back home, I unpacked the car, got Bob to bed for a nap, and put myself back in bed, exhausted. Although Bob's and my schedule went back to our usual routine, I felt sicker each day.

Finally, I gave up getting well on my own and made an appointment to see a doctor. My primary care doctor was on vacation, so I agreed to see another internist. At the beginning of the meeting, I gave her a quick sketch of my situation. I told her the details of the cold and mentioned that I was the caregiver for my husband who had Alzheimer's disease. She asked me a few questions, including, "How long have you been caregiving?"

"Seven years."

Next question: "Are you depressed?"

Unable to answer right away, I started to cry. Although I hadn't thought about depression, I now was struck by the realization I probably was depressed. Who wouldn't be, I said to myself.

She prescribed antibiotics after telling me I had bronchitis. And she prescribed an anti-depressant. I left her office feeling that someone had not only asked me how I was doing but also offered something to help. I felt better already.

Six months later, we tried another respite stay at the same facility which was not as successful. At the end of the stay, when I picked Bob up, he was out of sorts. He told me that the building was locked (a locked facility is standard for dementia care facilities) and he could not get out without setting off alarms, which he told me he had done several times. He couldn't understand what the alarm was for and why the security guard got mad at him. I tried to explain that the alarm was triggered when he opened the door to the lobby, but it made no sense to him.

Only then did I recall that I had not explained the concept of a locked facility to him, thinking he might worry about it or that he wouldn't be able to remember it anyway. In anger and frustration, he let me know he didn't like it there.

Some months later, I still worried that if something happened to me, I would have no place for Bob to stay. I located another facility to try in a county to the east of us. We did a tour of the building and grounds, met with the manager, did reference checks on their reputation, and everything seemed fine. Bob agreed to try a five-day visit at this place. It turned out to be even more unsatisfactory.

At the end of his stay, I found him in a television room, slumped in a chair, almost in a stupor. I reasoned that his recently increased anti-anxiety medication had been too much, and he was over-medicated and barely able to walk, even with the aid of his walker. I tried not to panic, but I had never seen him appear so lethargic.

The staff couldn't tell me anything about what had happened, and they had lost his glasses and some of his clothes. One caregiver casually explained that he had fallen out of bed, and they had put his mattress on the floor. I couldn't imagine how he would have been able to sleep in that situation, but he was too foggy to tell me anything. His loss of speech made me worry that he'd had a stroke. It took me half an hour to gather up his belongings with no assistance from the staff and help him to the car as he leaned precariously on his walker.

Earlier in the month, I had arranged for a routine CT scan appointment at Kaiser after the respite stay. As I got into the car, I calmed myself by remembering we were going to Kaiser, and I could take him to the ER after the scan if he had not improved by that time.

He was just as groggy after the scan, so we went to the ER. After four hours and numerous tests, the ER doctor pronounced Bob to be stroke-free and able to go home if he could walk. By this time, he was talking to me, and I could see how much better he was.

The doctor asked if I thought I could get him home by myself. I thought I could but asked, "Do you think that he is better now because his medication has had more than four hours to wear off?"

"I think it's highly likely. Would you like me to help you get to your car?"

At this point, I was grateful for the improvement in Bob, relieved there were no signs of a stroke, and appreciated the help the doctor offered—more than I had received at the respite facility.

Although I still didn't have a care plan for Bob should something happen to me, I had learned valuable information about dementia facilities. They are not prepared for short visits and are unable to provide appropriate care for someone whose behavior is unfamiliar to them. I felt lucky that Bob was open to the respite experiments and never took any of his frustrations out on me.

Accepting the reality that Bob's stays at a respite facility were no longer in my future, I focused on changing our weekends so they were not all caregiving. One day I had an idea. I remembered how much both Bob and I liked Jenny, a former employee at Adult Day. She now had children to look after, but I hoped she might take part of her weekend to work for us.

My thought was that she might agree to take Bob on a drive on Sundays. Being in the car was always soothing to him, and a drive was something he could look forward to. I talked with Bob about Jenny and my drive idea. He remembered her, even though he had not seen her in some time. He liked the idea—such a relief to me. I don't think I could have started with a stranger at this point. Also, she was familiar with dementia anxiety and knew Bob well. She had a fondness for him, and when I called her she readily agreed to help.

Jenny created a Sunday drive activity that he grew to love: drive to the top of Atlas Peak Road where her great-grandmother had a ranch, return to the valley floor where she took him to the same café for his favorite take-out chicken salad, return to our home to eat the lunch where everything was familiar, and finish the afternoon with a short drive on the other side of town to buy a frozen yogurt. The outing made Sundays fun for Bob. I treasured having most of Sunday afternoon for myself.

Some months into this Sunday schedule, Bob and I had a disagreement during the week about something inconsequential. For Bob it was serious, and he lost his patience with me and the discussion. Abruptly, he announced, "I want Jenny!" I was taken aback. His request was childlike and felt like rejection to me. I took a deep breath and vowed to not respond in kind. His demand for Jenny helped me realize how important his connection to her had become, and I was grateful for that. My weekends were less stressful with Jenny's help.

Part Seven

Late Stage Journeys

CHAPTER 33

Referral to Hospice

Bob began to suffer every day from bouts of anxiety in 2009. This agitation woke him in the middle of the night and stayed with him at Adult Day on a regular basis.

A major source of his anxiety in the afternoon involved taking the bus home. The Adult Day staff explained to me that his worry about catching the bus surfaced every day almost as soon as he finished lunch. He would go to the lobby area, sit next to the receptionist, and ask her repeatedly if his bus had arrived.

The compassionate and inventive staff anticipated this anxiety and developed a plan to set aside his coveted spinach salad almost as a dessert for him after lunch. Before he went to the lobby to check on his bus, a staff person would lead him to a quiet room where he could relax in private and enjoy his salad. Because he was a slow eater, it would keep him occupied until his bus arrived at 2:30.

That year, Bob's anxiety came on without warning and hung on like a bad cold. I was armed only with the anti-anxiety drug Ativan to give him. I also took him to a Kaiser psychiatrist who tried a variety of other anti-anxiety medications. None worked—some made him feel worse. He would awaken me in the middle of the night by going to the kitchen and opening and closing drawers. One night I found him eating one banana after another with the door to the deck half-way open.

In December, Sheila at Adult Day called and asked me to come in for an appointment. She had helped me many times but gave no hint as to the problem she wanted to discuss this time. I began to fear the worst. Being aware of the frustrations I was having with him at home, I could imagine they might be having worse problems with him during the day.

When Sheila greeted me, she said she wanted Bob to be a part of the meeting too. My mind raced as to what this might mean. I thought Bob may have created some problem with another participant or staff person, and she needed my help to resolve it. I couldn't have been more wrong.

After Sheila located him, she told us both, "Let's meet in my office. It will be quiet there." She spoke softly, describing her recent return from a leave of absence. "I noticed right away that Bob had changed during the time I was gone. I didn't want to alert you, Cheri, if I was wrong, so I continued to monitor his behavior for those first weeks I was back. I also talked with other staff members who had observed the same behavior changes that I had. He has reached a point where he needs someone with him most of the time." She then added, "We do not have the resources to provide a staff member for each participant."

During this disclosure, Sheila mostly spoke to me, but I could sense Bob felt included as he watched Sheila and listened intently. I was fairly certain, however, he had no idea what she was saying. She continued, "We want to make a recommendation to you, Cheri." I began to dread the next words; I feared she was about to announce that Bob needed to be placed in a dementia facility.

"We think it's time to ask Bob's primary care physician for a referral to hospice," she said. "We want to give you time to make this transition, Cheri. He can stay in Adult Day for a while longer if you want to search for other options."

I was immediately relieved he had not gotten into trouble. I was trying to process what Sheila had recommended. I had always thought hospice was only for people with six months to live. I certainly knew he was in the late stages of the disease, but I was surprised hospice might be an answer now. Sheila waited for me to gather myself. "You think he can qualify for hospice now?" I asked.

Adult Day was a part of Napa Valley Hospice, so I was confident Sheila knew what she was talking about. I had even attended classes given by hospice staff. I knew they didn't have a residential facility, so I wasn't worried about Bob having to go somewhere new. He could stay at home.

Sheila nodded. "A person with dementia who is in persistent decline can qualify for hospice services in the home." I later learned that might include a daily visit from a home healthcare worker, a nurse assigned to us, and volunteers to visit with Bob. He could continue to do at home whatever he was capable of. She continued, "They do not have to be six months away from the end. And as you probably know, hospice services are paid for by Medicare." (I recently learned that the "persistent decline" qualification for Medicare has changed—caregivers should check with their healthcare provider for current information.)

Sheila explained what would happen next: "Contact his primary care doctor and tell her you'd like a referral to hospice. You can tell her we have made this recommendation and are willing to share our records with her to help put together the necessary health information."

"We are Kaiser members, and I know they have their own hospice services," I said. "Could we request Napa Valley Hospice instead? It would be so much better for us as we are familiar with so many people here."

"I'm pretty sure it won't be a problem, especially if you tell Bob's doctor about the long-standing relationships you both have here," she answered. "Please alert your doctor that we will forward all the medical records we have on Bob." Then she stood up which I took as a signal that our meeting was concluded.

There was nothing more to do except to thank her and guide Bob toward the door. I could see Sheila was relieved at this outcome. It must have been difficult for her not knowing if I might get defensive and fight to keep Bob in the Adult Day program.

By the time our meeting ended, the program day was almost over. Sheila promised she would communicate Bob's departure to everyone. I thanked her with a small hug and guided Bob out the door.

In the car, he started asking questions right away. "What was that all about? I didn't know what she was talking about."

"Let's drive home, Bob. We can talk about it when we get there," I suggested. He seemed satisfied with that answer which gave me some time to process what had just transpired. The feelings of relief did not suddenly disappear, but I began to worry that I felt good about the hospice recommendation because it might be easier for me. I also realized I would never have to tell Bob he was moving to a dementia facility—my worst fear of all. He would be able to be home as his disease went into its final stages.

That afternoon I called Bob's primary care physician and left a message about needing a referral to hospice. Within the hour, I was talking with her about what needed to happen next. She saw the reasoning about referring Bob to Napa Valley Hospice and was pleased that Adult Day would forward his health records to her.

By the time I got off the phone, Bob had already gone to his bedroom to take his afternoon nap. I checked on him and then began to prepare dinner. It gave me time to think through how I would tell Bob what was about to take place in our lives.

After dinner, I brought up the topic. I couldn't tell if he remembered the meeting or not, but I had to start somewhere. "Remember the meeting we had today with Sheila?" I said.

"Yes, I know we met with her, but I couldn't follow what she was saying."

"She wanted to tell us Adult Day thinks you will now qualify for hospice, which means that you can stay at home from now on. I'm sorry you won't be able to go to Adult Day, but I think it's been getting harder and harder for you. Isn't that right?"

"Yeah," he said. "I have a lot of trouble with the bathroom and getting on and off the bus is hard too."

I told him I had started the process to get a referral to hospice. I couldn't tell how he felt about this news as I was struggling with my own feelings. I began to cry as I put my arms around him. I wanted to reassure him this was the best thing we could hope for. "I'm so relieved you will be able to be at home, sweetie. I've been worried about what we would do if you couldn't go to Adult Day anymore."

"I'm not sure I understand, but if you think it's the best thing, that makes me feel better," he managed to reply. This trust he had in me always gave me confidence and reminded me what a gentle guy he still was.

"We'll be seeing some of the same staff we got to know at Mind Boosters and Adult Day. And you'll be at home." I hoped that repeating the "at home" part of the news would be comforting. "Your doctor thought hospice nurses might come to our house tomorrow to begin to set everything up, so that's pretty quick. We can talk more about this when I know more."

"Okay," he said. "I think I want to go to bed now."

I felt he had been through enough for one day—both of us had. A short time later, I went to bed with the anticipation of a new beginning, but sadness had surfaced too. I knew Bob would miss attending Adult Day, and I would be giving up daily free time. That loss was minor in comparison to the relief I felt that a dementia facility was not going to be in our immediate future. The picture of having him safe at home relaxed me to the point that I fell asleep immediately. Sleep had been hard to come by in recent weeks.

CHAPTER 34

Our Hospice Experience

nlike what they say about justice, the wheels of Napa Valley Hospice moved quickly. Two days after my meeting with Sheila at Adult Day, two women who were Registered Nurses (RN) from hospice came to our home to do the admitting procedure. I thought admitting only happened at hospitals, so I was surprised at the amount of information they collected and the paperwork they required. They were kind and careful with me, clearly having experience with caregivers, especially those having cared for a person with dementia.

They told me I was to stop all of Bob's current medications. They then prescribed medicine appropriate for palliative care which they explained would provide relief from the symptoms of dementia. They also gave me pain medication, which he would need later.

They also ordered a hospital bed, a wheelchair, a moveable tray to fit over his bed, and other items to make him comfortable.

That afternoon, after they left, the doorbell unexpectedly rang. When I opened the door, a woman in an attractive uniform put out her hand and introduced herself. "Hi, I'm Bernie from hospice." She was energetic and seemed confident. I liked both qualities. She carried a large black bag full of what I soon learned were all the items she needed to do her job. She quickly explained she was our Home Health Aide and would be visiting three days a week to help care for Bob. I was not expecting anyone so soon but took her to Bob's bedroom where he was waking up from a nap. I introduced Bernie and reminded him we would have people from hospice coming to our house now.

She seemed to know exactly what to do to put him at ease. Bernie was also able to keep the conversation going as she explained everything she did while asking his permission, although he mostly said, "Yes" and "Okay," as she went about her tasks. It had been a couple of days since he had showered and shaved, so that's where she started. She knew how to bathe him in bed and wash his hair using shampoo and warm water. Shaving him with his electric razor was easy for her. I knew that with clean hair and a smooth face he would feel so much better, and he certainly seemed to.

Eventually, Bernie's visits were increased to five days a week. She always arrived at 9:30 a.m. I gave Bob his breakfast earlier so he was ready for her. Because of hospice policy, I wasn't able to leave the house until after she left, so I began to schedule client appointments for the afternoon. I had stopped looking for new consulting clients but still wanted to meet the expectations of my long-term clients. I knew there would be no charges for hospice services but having my consulting income allayed my fears about meeting unexpected expenses.

I was so grateful for Bernie's assistance. She taught me how to care for Bob at each stage, anticipating situations before I recognized them. She was smart and efficient. He usually wore a cotton knit turtleneck and sweatpants instead of pajamas since he usually complained of being cold. When it became too difficult for me to pull his turtleneck over his head—I felt I was almost strangling him—Bernie showed me how to cut the back open so I could easily put his arms through and then the neck wasn't a problem. His turtleneck became a hospital gown with a few snips of her scissors.

I was surprised at how compliant Bob was with her. He never said much, but I think he counted on me to be Bernie's partner and keep an eye on everything she did. Every other day, she changed Bob's clothes and his bed linens. I had more laundry than I'd ever had but having him in a clean bed made me feel as good as if I were the one getting newly changed bedsheets.

Within a week of Bob entering the hospice program, he fell several times when we were alone. After dinner, he would sometimes want to sit in the living room. Moving from the new hospice-ordered wheelchair to the couch seemed easy enough, but it was hard reversing the steps. This was often when he fell. In trying to help him up, I began to realize he hadn't fallen; he had collapsed. He tried to follow my instructions to get his legs underneath him to get up, but the brain/muscle connection was gone. I tried to reassure him it was all right, and I would get help.

Adult Day had given me a non-emergency number to call in case of a fall. The local fire department responded to the calls sans sirens. The fire truck came each time with guys in big firefighting gear. It usually took three of them to return Bob to bed. He looked so relieved to be back in bed and thanked the men in his gentlemanly way.

Isabella, the RN and leader of our hospice team, visited that first week too. She walked confidently into the house the first day and quickly explained to me what her role was. She would be visiting once a week but more often if needed. I liked her right away. I told her about Bob's collapsing, and she advised me to keep him in bed. "It's too dangerous to have him take the risk of getting up," she said, "only to fall and possibly break a bone or worse." Her suggestion made me feel like Bob's decline was on fast forward, but when I told him what she had said and saw how relieved he was about not getting up, I knew we were doing the right thing.

Isabella was great with Bob and could get him to laugh. She also nursed his soon-to-appear bedsores and trained me how to apply the medicine and change the bandages. I was nervous about getting the medicines applied and re-placing the dressings. Eventually, to Isabella's amazement, the sores healed. She told me she had never seen bed sores heal on a bed-bound person. I wasn't surprised — Bob's surgery incisions had also closed quickly and impressed the surgeon. I wondered, how could his skin have the power to heal when his brain couldn't make his body get up off the floor?

Every few weeks, Isabella was required to draw a sample of Bob's blood to make sure his decline was still, in hospice terminology, "persistent." I was warned each time if that were not the case he would "graduate from hospice." This meant no more services. I held my breath each time, as I couldn't imagine what I would do without all the help I now had.

Isabella explained to me that if I had any medical problems with Bob during the night, I could call the hospice night nurse. Thinking that was a great service, I never imagined I would need it until maybe the end. But one evening during Christmas week, in our first month with hospice, Bob became so restless and fearful I didn't know what to do. He seemed miserable but couldn't tell me what was wrong. Just before midnight, I finally called the night nurse number. The woman who answered reassured me she would be there in 30 minutes. Indeed, within that time, I heard her car pull into the driveway. I opened the front door and saw a slight woman in a long cape get out of the car. As she walked up the sidewalk, she smiled. I knew an angel had arrived.

She examined Bob and reassured me he was all right but that he was probably feeling both anxiety and pain. She suggested a medicine that would help both symptoms. She had it in her bag and explained it was my decision to start him on it or not. We talked about what it would and wouldn't do. She explained that starting pain meds early is best so the pain doesn't get a head start. I was afraid of side effects, especially hallucinations. She reassured me that was not common with this drug and stayed with me until I felt confident about making the decision. I finally decided we would start him on the drug, thankful she had helped me make such an important decision. Fortunately, it did not cause him hallucinations.

To my surprise, after already receiving a lot of help from hospice, their volunteer coordinator called to ask if I was interested in having volunteers visit Bob. When other hospice staff visited, I was not allowed to leave the house. This was different, she explained. I could leave for a couple of hours while Bob was with the volunteer. I immediately said yes. I was able to have two volunteer visits a week and could specify what might be most helpful to Bob. I knew he would like a male visitor, so I asked if it was possible to specify gender. It was. I also asked if anyone played music for patients. The coordinator then arranged for a former professional musician to come every week. He played the guitar and mandolin. Bob could not carry on a conversation anymore, but I could tell the music soothed him.

The other part of our professional hospice team consisted of a social worker and a chaplain. They were each available on a weekly basis if I wanted. The first chaplain, named Patrick, was a big man who was gentle and caring. He would visit with Bob for a few minutes, reading or singing to him. After visiting with Bob, he would come into the living room to see me. I sensed he was ministering to us both. When I asked how he thought Bob was, he would say, "He's not ready to go." I was relieved to hear his assessment.

A few months later, Patrick took another job and left the Napa Valley. I was sorry to see him leave, but his replacement was a woman, also kind and gentle. She apologized for the change but made it easy for me to open up to her, as if she knew all that had transpired with Bob. She was younger than I, (as most of the staff were), with a soft voice and an approachable manner. She too, would visit Bob first and then spend time with me.

The social worker was an enormous help to me. Gina was trained in all aspects of death and dying. She listened carefully to my questions and was always supportive in her answers. At the end of our first meeting, I asked if I could see her again.

"Of course," she said. "Most people only want to ask me questions about final arrangements, so they're usually content with one visit."

I explained I had no family in the area and would like to see her once a week. Agreed. We never ran out of things to talk about. As Bob's condition changed, and I began to see final steps in his decline, she was able to help me understand the process he was going through.

For months, I had been worried about the responsibilities of appropriately managing the end of Bob's life. He had agreed to a brain autopsy at the request of the Alzheimer's Disease Center. It was up to me to meet this obligation. I knew I needed to alert the Center when he passed, but I was unsure about everything else. It was Gina who guided me through the communication I needed to do in advance with the Center. Once I learned where and when to call at the end, who would come for Bob, and where they would take him, I began to find some peace in facing the end.

As soon the hospice team was organized and scheduled, I had time to think about what else we might need since Bob became bedbound. My mind went to Rudy who had been so good with Bob in the early days. I called Rudy, asked him if he could work with us again. Our plan to engage him early, in case we needed him later, turned out to be one of the few things I was truly successful at planning. I rehired him to come for five hours a day, four days a week. At his first visit, Rudy hugged me as soon as he came in the front door. When I took him back to see Bob, Bob's face lit up with a big smile and Rudy hugged him. Rudy was a Certified Nursing Assistant (CNA) and his prior experience of caring for bedridden patients was valuable now. He also taught me how to move a person in bed so I wouldn't hurt myself. It gave me such a sense of relief to know Rudy would be with us to help. He also prepared and fed Bob lunch and dinner each day.

During that last year, despite all the help, there were still many tasks that fell to me, including my consulting work. I was tired all the time. Only through Rudy's help was I able to take a nap in the middle of the day to give me an energy boost for the rest of the day and evening.

One day when I awoke from my nap, I went to see if Rudy had fed Bob his lunch. Bob was asleep, but Rudy gave me an update. Earlier, he had been looking at Bob when he awakened. Rudy said Bob looked right at him and said, "Hi, sweetie heartie." Rudy thought it was great, explaining that if Bob was talking maybe he wasn't as bad as I thought. I agreed that the talking was good news, but I also had an awareness for the first time what it really meant; Bob had confused Rudy with me. The sweetie heartie was an old joke between us. I had to accept that Bob probably didn't know who I was anymore. Nonetheless, I thanked Rudy for passing on the story. He paid such close attention to Bob; I had to be grateful.

While hospice was my main support system during Bob's last year, others made his last months easier. Chris, who had cooked for us over the years of Bob's illness, continued to provide a meal once a week. My neighbor, Teresa, volunteered to sit with Bob when I had an unexpected need to be somewhere but no time to arrange for a paid caregiver.

When Bob became bedbound, it never occurred to me that he would be in bed so long that his hair would need to be cut. Bernie shaved him every morning and washed his hair, but of course, it continued to grow. Not keeping a secret about Bob's illness made it easier to ask my hairstylist for help. She wasn't surprised when I asked if she could come to our house and give Bob a haircut. She enthusiastically said, "Of course! I'll come on Sunday." Learning to ask for help was getting easier, and her upbeat response, like other people, made me feel glad that I had asked.

I alerted Bob on Sunday morning that he was going to have his hair cut that day. He smiled at me, but I was sure he didn't know what I had said. Nonetheless, I felt like I was still keeping him appraised of what was happening. Jill had difficulty getting to the back of Bob's head and eventually crawled up on the bedframe from behind him (where the bed was tilted up). We laughed as she climbed up the frame of the bed. "It's good I used to be a gymnast," she said, "so I can do haircuts like this." I couldn't imagine Bob's former barber crawling around Bob's body.

In May of that year, 2010, I learned from a woman in my support group about the Threshold Choir. Around the world, Threshold Choirs sing *a cappella* in small groups to people at the threshold of their lives. The description of their music sounded like it could be an unusual spiritual experience for both Bob and me. I made arrangements for the Napa Threshold Choir to visit Bob on a Friday afternoon.

Friday afternoon at 4:00 came soon enough. When the doorbell rang, I opened our front door to four smiling women, all clearly experienced with such visits. After I invited them in and we introduced ourselves, I soon realized I had met a couple of them at other times and in other circumstances. Their quiet friendliness made their presence easy from the start.

I took them to Bob's bedroom, introducing them by simply saying, "These women have come to sing for you, Bob." They gathered around his bed in a semi-circle, not too close, but not too far away, either. I'll never forget that their first song started with the phrase, "I will sing for you, my friend." Their unaccompanied voices were clear but soft and seemed to surround us with loving care. They sang for about 30 minutes. Many songs brought me to tears. When I looked at Bob, I had the sense he took it all in, his eyes fixing on one singer and then another. Usually, he went to sleep when visitors came. This time he was fully present.

When I walked the singers to the door, they said they would be happy to come back and sing on Fridays. I was delighted. Caregiving can be so lonely; I was already looking forward to having the choir be part of our weekly routine.

When people ask, "How did you do it?" referring to the nine years of Bob's illness and how long I was his care-giver, I tell them I learned to ask for help, starting with Rudy. When Bob's last year came, I welcomed hospice and others who had become a part of our team. Our last year together was not the hardest. Yes, there were days I didn't want anybody to come to our house; I missed my privacy and desperately needed rest. I would not have been able to make it through that last year without all the care and support both Bob and I received from our hospice team and the friends and neighbors who had helped from the beginning.

CHAPTER 35

My Morning Farewell

Bob died in the early morning of February 8, 2011. I had checked on him at 3:30 a.m. as I routinely did to administer more pain medication. He was sound asleep then, but I was able to insert the hypodermic with medication (without the needle of course) into his mouth to keep him from pain during the balance of the night. When I awakened at 6:00 in the morning and went into his room, he had left this world.

I was comforted by the memory that I had told him good-bye like I did every night since he had stopped eating. In the last months, while he could still talk he expressed his concern about me after he was no longer alive. I never knew what specifically he was worried about; by then, he wasn't able to communicate complicated feelings. My frequent response to him had become almost an affirmation for me: "I'll be all right, sweetheart. I will miss you and think about you every day. We have enough resources to take care of me, and there is nothing for you to worry about. I love you."

Sometimes I would almost start to cry before I finished. I kissed him on the cheek and left the room hoping the words were floating about and would find their way to his ears.

On this morning, I knew I had additional responsibilities. Keeping my emotions at bay, I was aware that timeliness was important. I called hospice right away, then the Alzheimer's Disease Center number I had been given, and then I waited for the Center's transportation service to arrive to take Bob to Sacramento for the autopsy. I was numb and exhausted.

Hospice staff had prepared me well for this morning. They explained their organization had the authority to pronounce a person dead—contacting a coroner was not necessary. After making those two calls, I returned to Bob's bedroom and stood by his bed in a dazed state. Hospice arrived in less than 15 minutes. They embraced me at our front door, and I felt comforted by their presence. I was grateful they were there to take charge of whatever needed to be done. When the transportation service arrived, they transferred Bob to a gurney, then wrapped him in a sheet, his face thus gone from view. They wheeled the gurney to the front door and left within minutes.

Although I was on automatic pilot, I managed to say thank you to the hospice team as I showed them to the door. Then I was all alone.

Feeling both enervated and numb, I walked down the hall to my office and started making phone calls to family members. Eventually, at 10:00 a.m. I went back to my bed, the only place I wanted to be. I couldn't sleep but knew the world had changed and began to sense a void I couldn't yet comprehend. Having years of advance notice of Bob's impending death did little to help me prepare for it.

In those first few days, I could see that living without Bob, even a very ill Bob, was going to be another difficult stage in this seemingly endless Alzheimer's journey. The relief I had imagined was yet to come.

Some weeks later, I contacted the grief services staff at hospice but I didn't sign up. I learned about the service choices and the meeting schedule. Attending a grief group would have to wait. I had learned that burnout from caregiving has a long recovery time. I had felt burnout for a long time. I gave myself time to do nothing which felt selfish, but at some level I knew it was the right thing to do for me.

Three months later, I found my way to a grief group for men and women. It was held in the same building where I had taken Bob to his beloved Mind Boosters and later Adult Day. It was an odd sensation to be there without Bob. I was pleased to be in a space that felt familiar, but it would take me a long time to become accustomed to being alone in places where we had frequently been a couple.

My eventual anchor at Napa Valley Hospice was its women's grief group which met once a week, facilitated by a specialist in grief matters. Slowly, the void I experienced that first morning began to fade as I finally let myself feel the loss of Bob and my life with him. The friends I made at the group helped me then and also today; I still see the women, now my friends, regularly for lunch.

Hospice's grief group proved to be the final example of how support groups are the best that healthcare has to offer Alzheimer's patients, their families, and caregivers. As one expression of my gratitude, I began work as a hospice volunteer, recording patients' favorite stories from their lives as keepsakes for their families.

Epilogue

In May of 2011, I received a warm yet technical letter from the Director of the Alzheimer's Disease Center at UC Davis. He started with a genuine thank you for our agreeing to the autopsy and assured me that their findings from the autopsy had helped the University in their research.

The conclusion, however, was as confusing as Bob's years of illness. The autopsy had established that he had three diseases: normal pressure hydrocephalus (the reason he had the shunt put in), cerebrovascular dementia and, yes, Alzheimer's. The last sentence in the letter partially explained why Bob had received so little help from the medical profession: "This is a complex case, both clinically and pathologically."

I already knew there was no cure for Alzheimer's disease, but I had hoped the autopsy might give some hints as to why healthy Bob was one of its innocent victims. He would have been relieved to learn that there was nothing he should have done that he didn't. No suggestions of poor diet, lack of exercise, or poor mental fitness. I read between

the lines: His vulnerability to the three causes of his dementia will remain a mystery.

I mailed copies of the autopsy results to Bob's adult children. And I tried to stop asking the universe, "Why did this
happen to Bob?"

Note to Readers

There are numerous websites about dementia-related diseases and caregiver information. The Alzheimer's Association website (*alz.org*) has the most complete website for caregivers.

The Napa Valley Hospice and Adult Day Services has changed its name to Collabria Care (*collabriacare.org*). It is still the home of Mind Boosters, Adult Day, and Hospice programs.

CPSIA information can be obtained
at www.ICGtesting.com
Printed in the USA
FSHW010838260720
72482FS